GERIATRIC
RESPIRATORY
CARE

D1468154

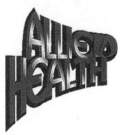

GERIATRIC RESPIRATORY CARE

Helen M. Sorenson, B.A., R.R.T.
Director of Clinical Education in Respiratory Therapy
Metropolitan Community College
Omaha, Nebraska

James A. Thorson, Ed.D.
Professor and Chairman
Department of Gerontology
University of Nebraska at Omaha
Omaha, Nebraska

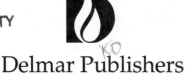

Delmar Publishers

an International Thomson Publishing company I(T)P®

Albany • Bonn • Boston • Cincinnati • Detroit • London • Madrid
Melbourne • Mexico City • New York • Pacific Grove • Paris • San Francisco
Singapore • Tokyo • Toronto • Washington

NOTICE TO THE READER

Cover Design: Brian Sullivan

Delmar Staff

Publisher: Susan Simpfenderfer
Acquisitions Editor: Dawn Gerrain
Developmental Editor: Debra Flis
Project Editor: Elizabeth LaManna
Production Coordinator: John Mickelbank
Art and Design Coordinator: Vincent S. Berger
Editorial Assistant: Donna L. Leto

COPYRIGHT © 1998
By Delmar Publishers, Inc.
an International Thomson Publishing Company

The ITP logo is a trademark under license.

Printed in the United States of America

For more information, contact:

Delmar Publishers
3 Columbia Circle, Box 15015
Albany, NY 12212-5015

International Thomson Publishing Europe
Berkshire House 168-173
High Holborn
London, WC1V7AA
England

Thomas Nelson Australia
102 Dodds Street
South Melbourne, 3205
Victoria, Australia

Nelson Canada
1120 Birchmount Road
Scarborough, Ontario
Canada, M1K 5G4

International Thomson Editores
Campos Eliseos 385, Piso 7
Col Polanco
11560 Mexico D F Mexico

International Thomson Publishing Gmbh
Königswinterer Strasse 418
53227 Bonn
Germany

International Thomson Publishing Asia
221 Henderson Road #05-10
Henderson Building
Singapore 0315

International Thomson Publishing - Japan
Hirakawacho Kyowa Building, 3F
2-2-1 Hirakawacho
Chiyoda-ku, 102 Tokyo
Japan

1 2 3 4 5 6 7 8 9 10 XXX 02 01 00 99 98 97 96

Library of Congress Cataloging-in-Publication Data

Sorenson, Helen M.
Geriatric respiratory care / Helen M. Sorenson, James A. Thorson.
    p.   cm.
Includes bibliographical references and index.
ISBN 0–8273–7054–7
1. Aged—Medical care. 2. Aging. 3. Respiratory diseases in old age. 4. Respiratory therapy. 5. Geriatrics. 6. Respiratory organs—Aging. I. Thorson, James A., 1946– . II. Title.
[DNLM: 1. Respiratory Therapy—in old age. 2. Geriatrics. WB 342 S713g 1997]
RC952.S67   1997
618.97—dc21
DNLM/DLC
for Library of Congress   97–9709
                                                     CIP

CONTENTS

PREFACE

The graying of America that has been observed during the final decades of the twentieth century will accelerate during the beginning years of the twenty-first century. Baby boomers will begin to retire and there will be unprecedented pressures on the health care system. Acute and chronic care facilities and programs are currently being extended by subacute and home care agencies and institutions. These trends will continue. The need for health care professionals who are knowledgeable about aging and about aged people will be critical in future years.

Health care professions, nursing and medicine in particular, have begun to respond to this demographic revolution. Unfortunately, allied health professions have been slow to integrate geriatrics into their curricula. We believe that this text is the first in gerontology and geriatrics focused entirely on respiratory care. It is meant to serve a number of purposes. No doubt it will be used in some innovative programs that develop a freestanding course in geriatric respiratory care. Others may find it useful as a text for a section of another course, on home health care, for example. It may also be used as the foundation for continuing professional education programs. In whatever ways the book is used, it is our hope that it ultimately will be of benefit to older adults and to the health care practitioners who care for them.

In this text, psychological and social aspects of gerontology and clinical aspects of geriatrics are combined in the various chapters. Taking the care of the aged in perspective, it is emphasized that personal and subjective relationships may often be as important as technical proficiency. Chapter 1 examines the aging processes, the aging of the population, and the emergence of universal chronic illness. A section on developing approaches to rapport with older people is also included. Chapter 2 assesses various theories of gerontology and issues in adult socialization. Chapter 2 also discusses the psychological aspects of gerontology, including development and continuity across the life span as well as emotional illness and dementia. Suggestions are given on dealing with cognitively impaired older adults.

Chapter 3 addresses the biological causes of aging, including theories of physical aging and an overview of physical changes, morbidity, and mortality. Pulmonary changes associated with the aging process and implications are examined. Aging is characterized by gradual decline and chronicity; many health care professionals are focused on the cure of acute conditions and may need to gain a different perspective when dealing with the illnesses associated with old age. In Chapter 4, cardiac, cerebrovascular, and restrictive lung diseases are examined, as well as cancer and tuberculosis.

Chapter 5 provides extensive coverage of pharmacology, including successful drug therapy, pharmacokinetics, pharmacodynamics, and adverse drug reactions.

Chapter 6 is an examination of acute diseases and their presentation in later life, including acute cardiovascular and acute respiratory diagnoses, hypothermia, and an extensive treatment of postoperative complications.

Chapter 7 discusses the issues of long-term care at home and within skilled and intermediate care institutions. In particular, the social message of institutionalization is emphasized, with its implication that entry into a nursing home may be interpreted by older people as a one-way trip without hope of discharge. Compassionate care and palliative measures are emphasized. Home care and promoting independence outside of institutions is also covered. Chapter 8 provides an in-depth discussion on the end of life, including the demographics of life and death, coverage of types of death, and quality of life issues. Special emphasis is placed on advance directives, including living wills and durable power of attorney for health care. The issue of termination of life support, ethical decision making, weaning terminally ill patients from mechanical ventilation, and suicide, an exceedingly important issue among older people, is also covered.

Overall, the goal with this first book on geriatric respiratory care is to integrate the social with the technical. While various health conditions present differently in later life, caring for older people as individuals is also important. Issues in the lives of older people have important outcomes in their wellness and in their willingness to survive. Our hope is that the care of older people is characterized by tenderness, patience, and warmth.

ACKNOWLEDGMENTS

The authors and Delmar staff wish to thank the following reviewers:

Elaine K. Allen, BA, RRT, RPFT
Program Director
Respiratory Care
Thiel College
Greenville, Pennsylvania

Allen W. Barbaro, MS, RRT
Program Director
Respiratory Care Program
Collin County Community College
McKinney, Texas

Deborah L. Cullen, EdD, RRT
Professor and Director
Respiratory Therapy Program
Indiana University
Indianapolis, Indiana

Beverly Edwards, BHS, RRT
Program Director
Respiratory Care Program
Florida Community College at Jay
Jay, Florida

*Dedicated to the
memory of
our parents*

CHAPTER ONE

GERONTOLOGY: THE STUDY OF AGING

KEY TERMS

ageism
compression of morbidity
demography
empathy

epidemiology
geriatrics
gerontology
life expectancy

life span
locus of control
rectangular survival curve

LEARNING OBJECTIVES

After completing this chapter, the reader should be able to:

1. Describe how gerontology differs from geriatrics.
2. List several ways that people age at different rates.
3. Give examples of how the population is aging.
4. Provide several of the correlates of longevity.
5. Explain some important approaches to rapport with older people.

INTRODUCTION

Older people are major consumers of health care services. They are frequently cared for by professionals in the field of respiratory care, who confront chronic health problems on a daily basis. The elderly have the greatest need for the services of the respiratory care practitioner.

This chapter looks at aging as a process, not an event, and it explores the concept of aging at different rates. It reviews demographics of an aging population and the emergence of universal chronic illness. The differences between **life span** and **life expectancy** are discussed. The chapter concludes with advice on communicating with older people and helping them maintain internal control.

THE MULTIDISCIPLINARY NATURE OF GERONTOLOGY AND GERIATRICS

Gerontology, the study of the aging process, is the scientific foundation for **geriatrics,** the clinical management and treatment of older persons. Both gerontology and geriatrics are multidisciplinary. The field of gerontology is made up of research from biology, psychology, sociology, economics, and other disciplines. Practitioners from medicine, nursing, respiratory care, social work, physical therapy, and other allied health fields all make contributions to geriatrics. The respiratory care practitioner is a member of a multidisciplinary team. In the therapeutic setting, there are many professionals who have a role in the care of the aged. No one profession can claim to have primary importance. The hospital chaplain may provide care that is seen by the older patient as equally important as the care provided by the physician. As the roles and importance of different professionals vary in the care of older people, so do the needs and wants of older people. Thus, all of the members of the health care team need to gain knowledge in the study of aging.

CARE OF THE AGED IN PERSPECTIVE

As the importance of respiratory care is put into context in the treatment of the aged, the study of aging itself should be put into perspective as well.

AGING AS A PROCESS

No one simply becomes old. That is, aging is a process rather than an event. People do not cross a particular threshold and suddenly arrive at old age. The aging process is gradual, cumulative, and inevitable for those who live long enough. The commonly accepted definition of 65 as the beginning of old age is false. In 1884, Chancellor Otto von Bismarck of Germany picked 65 as the age at which civil servants could begin receiving pensions. Lacking a better precedent, the U.S. Congress in 1935 took age 65 as the starting point for the Social Security program (Thorson, 1995). Government programs need a set point for their beginning, but these points are often arbitrary.

Sixty-five may not be an exact beginning of old age for anyone. There are many vital, active people who are doing exciting things well into their eighties (Figure 1-1). On the other hand, therapists frequently confront patients in their fifties and sixties who seem to be old.

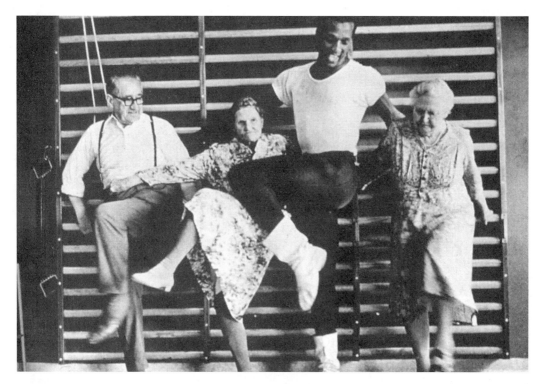

Figure 1-1 *Old age and retirement are a time of satisfaction and growth for most people.*

AGING AT DIFFERENT RATES

People age at different rates. Not only do people arrive at old age at different times but different organs and systems age at different rates as well. Variations may be due to genetics or environmental effects. Hearing is a sense that peaks in efficiency at about age 10 and then begins a gradual decline throughout the rest of life. No 20-year-old has hearing as acute as a 10-year-old. Hearing is one of the physical capacities that does not improve or respond to exercise. There is no therapy that can make it better. The best alternative is to preserve it. Those who are exposed to prolonged, damaging noise in a sense have old hearing. A rock musician might easily have the heart and lungs of a 25-year-old but the hearing ability of a 55-year-old. People with Alzheimer's disease may have brain impairments but essentially healthy circulatory systems. It might be said that smokers have old lungs. Many older people have arthritis that limits their daily activities, making them act old even if they are relatively healthy in other ways.

As a practical matter, however, most people age at a fairly constant rate, but it is quite possible to have chronic health problems within one bodily system earlier than another. This situation is fairly typical. The circulatory system might show serious problems while the nervous system is still relatively intact. However, it should be remembered that systems affect the functioning of each other. Declines in one may well precipitate declines in others. Diabetes, for example, has important influences on declining abilities in other systems.

INTERRELATIONSHIP OF SOCIAL, PSYCHOLOGICAL, AND PHYSICAL ASPECTS OF AGING

Psychological, social, and physical aspects of aging are connected. Depression, a psychological problem, and poverty, a social problem, may each have important outcomes in terms of poor nutrition, for example. Limited intake of necessary nutrients might then result in physical health problems. Arthritis, a physical problem, often limits ability to get around. It is not uncommon to find arthritic older people who are dehydrated because obtaining fluids may require walking to the kitchen. Dehydration in the aged commonly is associated with delirium. Thus, it could be said that a physical problem, arthritis, may be the underlying cause for an acute confusional state brought on by dehydration.

It therefore becomes important to assess older people's social and psychological state in addition to their physical well-being. Because older people have less marginal capacity in many different areas, they are more likely to experience decline in one realm that has been precipitated by decline in another. What the sociologist has to say about aging may be of as much importance as what the biologist or the psychologist brings to the study of aging.

DEMOGRAPHICS OF AGING

Demography is the statistical study of human populations. It is usually thought of as a specialty area within sociology. The principal source of most demographic information is census data. The federal government, however, has other reporting units in addition to the Bureau of the Census. The National Center for Health Statistics, a unit of the Centers for Disease Control, is an example of another reporting body that gives epidemiological (literally, the study of epidemics) statistical data. **Epidemiology** tracks morbidity within populations. Various life insurance companies are also good sources of data on health and longevity. Together, these sources help to provide a demographic profile of the older population: how large it is, how it is growing, what illnesses and disabilities older people have, and the causes of death at different ages.

There are three basic elements of demography: immigration, birth rate, and mortality. Immigration and birth rate are often ignored and mortality is overemphasized when speaking of the older population. The average population age of a state or country has to do with in-migration and out-migration of young people and with how many people are born there, as well as how long people live.

For example, the United States has an increasing median age not only because people die later in life than was the case years ago but also because the birth rate began to decline in 1960 when birth control pills were first introduced (Thorson, 1995). Fewer babies equals an older population, on the average. A population trend in the opposite direction, however, is caused by in-migration. Most immigrants are young people. In contrast, many states with high percentages of old people have experienced the out-migration of their younger citizens. These factors all need to be examined when describing demographic trends.

Misinterpretations of longevity data are common. One popular expression is that, "Many people are living longer," inferring that increased longevity in the population is explained by lower mortality rates later in life. This is not precisely the case. A more correct way of explaining the increase of the older population would be to say that a greater proportion of the population is living long enough to become old. That is, the growth of the older population is not dependent on people living to very great ages so much as it is dependent on an increasing percentage of the population surviving into middle age. The average life expectancy increases because fewer people are dying at young ages. Thus, more people survive into later adulthood.

A GROWING AGING POPULATION

The proportion of the total U.S. population that is aged has grown rapidly within recent years. Within the older population, the oldest old (those 85 and older) is the fastest growing (Table 1-1).

In 1900, there were 3,080,000 people age 65 and older in the United States, representing 4.1 percent of the total population. Recall that birth rate and immigration, as well as

TABLE 1-1   Growth of the Older Population (in thousands), 1900–2050

Year	Total (all ages)	65 Years and Over		85 Years and Over	
		Number	**Percent**	**Number**	**Percent**
1900	75,995	3,080	4.1	122	0.2
1910	91,972	3,949	4.3	167	0.2
1920	105,711	4,933	4.7	210	0.2
1930	122,775	6,634	5.4	272	0.2
1940	131,669	9,019	6.8	365	0.3
1950	150,697	12,269	8.1	577	0.4
1960	179,323	16,560	9.2	929	0.5
1970	203,302	19,980	9.8	1,409	0.7
1980	226,546	25,550	11.3	2,240	1.0
1990	248,710	31,079	12.5	3,021	1.2
2000	268,266	34,882	13.0	4,622	1.7
2010	282,575	39,362	13.9	6,115	2.2
2020	294,364	52,067	17.7	6,651	2.3
2030	300,629	65,604	21.8	8,129	2.7
2040	301,807	68,109	22.6	12,251	4.1
2050	299,849	68,532	22.9	15,287	5.1

Note: *Data for 1900 to 1990 are census figures. Data for 2000 to 2050 are Middle Series census projections.*

Source: *U.S. Bureau of the Census. Current Population Reports, Special Studies, P23-178, Sixty-Five Plus in America. U.S. Government Printing Office. Washington, DC, 1992.*

mortality, play a part in demography. In 1900, both the birth rate and U.S. in-migration were high, which partly explains the relatively small percentage of the whole represented by older people at the beginning of the century.

There were only 122,000 people age 85 and older in 1900, representing just two-tenths of 1 percent of the population. By the end of the century, this group of the oldest old represents more than 4 million people, 1.7 percent of the total.

The older population has grown in two ways: in absolute numbers and as a proportion of the population as a whole. The number of people 65 years and older has increased ten times from a little over 3 million in 1900 to almost 35 million by the year 2000. The rate of those age 85 and older has increased more than twenty-six times in the twentieth century, from 122,000 to over 4,600,000. By the middle of the twenty-first century, those 85 and older will have grown to 5.1 percent of the total population.

BABY BOOMERS

Between 1990 and 2000, the growth of the group 65 years of age and older has been fairly small (Table 1-1). It is much less than the growth of the population age 65+ in the 1980s. Why was the group becoming 65 in the 1990s so much smaller? Most of these people were born during the years of the Great Depression (1929–1940) when the birth rate was unusually low. The growth in the older population that is projected to occur between the years 2010 and 2020 is a whopping 12.7 million more older people. This growth is explained by the postwar baby boom, when the number of births dramatically increased between 1946 and 1960. By the year 2011, the first of these baby boomers will become senior citizens. Those born in 1946 will then be 65; in 2031, the first of the baby boomers will turn 85.

The profile of the oldest old will change because of this influence of changes in the birth rate that took place 85 years previously. The relatively small cohort born during the Depression, all of whom will be 80+ by the year 2020, will die and be replaced by post–World War II baby boomers. Thus, the proportion of the population represented by the oldest old will take a dramatic jump between the years 2030 and 2040.

There is a bulge in the population figures represented by the postwar baby boomers that is not followed by those born in succeeding decades. Therefore, the new 65-year-olds in 2040 and 2050 will not be much larger than the groups that came before them.

IMPLICATIONS

There are some important practical outcomes that will be influenced by these demographic changes. The most obvious is the changes needed in the Social Security program. As more people grow into later adulthood and retire, there will be greater pressure on those who remain in the workforce to generate retirement income for their seniors.

Less noticeable will be the gradual changes that take place in the society as it moves from a culture where most people are young to a culture where more and more people are old. Parent care is already becoming an important issue. People who are themselves senior citizens are often involved in the care of very old people. There are many people in their seventies whose principal problem is care of parents in their nineties. The demographic trends show that this social issue will continue to gain importance.

As a greater amount of public benefits goes toward income maintenance and medical care for the aged, and more people have caregiving responsibilities for the very aged, some have predicted that there will be an increasing resentment among younger people. Generational conflict may increase in future years (Minkler and Robertson, 1991).

Home health care and institutional care of the aged will assume increasing importance and demand more and more practitioners. Needs for long-term care and subacute care will grow. It is likely that there will be labor shortages among therapists and clinicians who care for the aged.

THE EMERGENCE OF UNIVERSAL CHRONIC ILLNESS

The increase of the aged population will mean an increase in the need for health care practitioners. There is an additional concept that goes beyond the numbers of older people now and in the future, though. The aging population is itself aging. In the 1970s, about two-thirds of all of those 65 years and older were between 65 and 74 (Thorson, 1995). These younger elders as a group have relatively fewer health problems (Figure 1-2). Those age 75 and above, who have more chronic health problems, represented only about one-third of

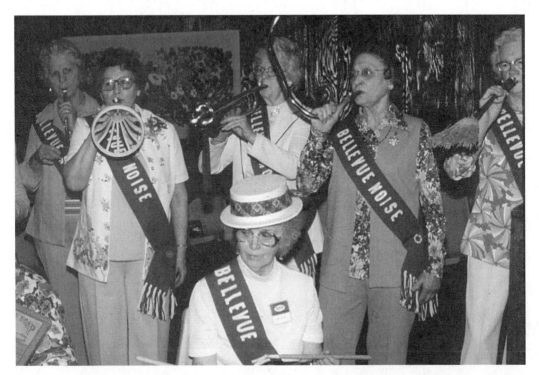

Figure 1-2 *The young old have fewer of the physical problems usually associated with old age.*

the total older population. Soon, those 75 and older will represent two-thirds of the elderly population. The implication is that there will be more frail and disabled people among the aged population and more people with chronic illness.

RECTANGULARIZATION OF THE SURVIVAL CURVE

The outcome of this demographic change was first described by two Stanford geriatricians, James F. Fries and Lawrence M. Crapo (1981). They pointed to the increasing number and proportion of the population reaching great ages and predicted a phenomenon that has increasingly come to pass: the emergence of universal chronic illness.

The curve represented by the percentage of survivors at particular ages has become more steep in recent years (Figure 1-3). This **rectangular survival curve** demonstrates that fewer people are dying in childhood and young adulthood. Fries and Crapo predict that this trend will continue. With good health care, most people may be able to anticipate about 85 years of disability-free life. With the conquest of communicable, acute illness, however, has come the emergence of universal chronic illness. People no longer die of childhood dis-

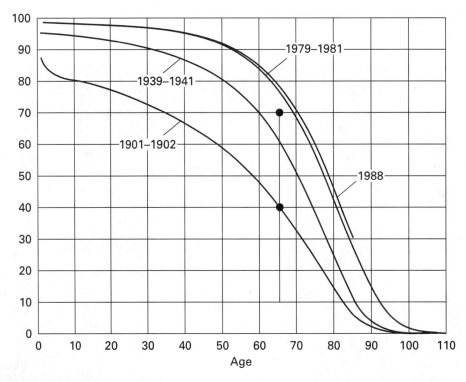

Figure 1-3 *Percentage of persons surviving to each age according to life tables for United States, 1900–1988. (Source: U.S. Bureau of the Census. Current Population Reports, Special Studies, P23–178, Sixty-Five Plus in America. Washington, DC: U.S. Government Printing Office, 1992.)*

eases such as measles and diphtheria; they now live long enough to die from cancer or heart disease. There is a corresponding **compression of morbidity,** in that the last few years of life are likely to represent the accumulation of chronic illnesses and disability.

LIFE SPAN AND LIFE EXPECTANCY

It is common to confuse **life expectancy** (the average from a particular point, such as life expectancy at birth or life expectancy at age 65) with **life span** (the maximum for the species). The life span of humans is about 110 or 115 years, although hardly anyone reaches this outside limit (Thorson, 1995). Perhaps with genetic engineering the biological limit to life span may be extended in years to come. Still, few will reach the limit. As a practical matter, most people will die somewhere between their seventieth and their ninetieth years. Currently, the average life expectancy for a 65-year-old male is an additional 15.6 years; for a 65-year-old female it is an additional 18.9 years (National Center for Health Statistics, 1996). Life expectancy varies according to gender, health, race, and social status.

There are several correlates of longevity. In general, women live about 10 percent longer than men. At younger ages, whites and Asians have a greater life expectancy than blacks; however, this evens out by later life. People of higher socioeconomic status live longer than those who are poor. Another correlate of longevity is health. Those who are in poor health have poorer odds. The same is true of social networks. Those who have intimate companionship have better mortality experience than those who do not (Figure 1-4). Married

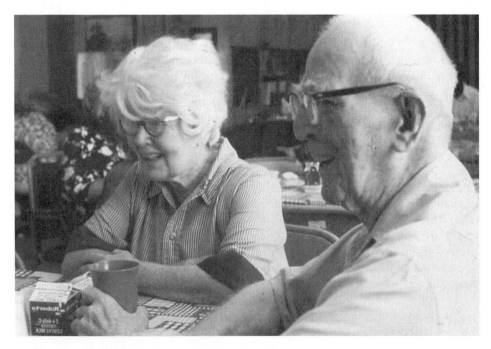

Figure 1-4 *An intact social network is a correlate of longevity.*

persons are lower in almost all causes of death than single, widowed, or divorced people (Thorson, 1995).

However the life expectancy varies, the life span and the overall rate of aging have remained relatively constant. Examples from literature confirm that "old" meant someone past the sixth decade of life even many years ago. For instance, in the Bible, Psalm 90 says, "The days of our lives are three score and ten years, or four score by reason of strength." In other words, more than 3,000 years ago the length of life was thought to be 70 or 80 years. This has not changed all that much. What has changed is the percentage of people in modern times who survive into old age.

ESTABLISHING RAPPORT WITH THE ELDERLY

Communicating and establishing rapport with the elderly is increasingly important for all health care professionals. Younger people in particular have been segregated from the elderly in present-day society. It would be fair to say that many people associate aging with death. Since most of the people who die are elderly, aging implies dissolution and death. The popular connection of aging with chronic illness and death may engender prejudice against the aged.

AGEISM

Perhaps the connection of aging with death partly explains the popular mania to postpone aging at all costs—having cosmetic surgery to remove signs of the aging process, dieting and eating health foods, going to fitness centers, and in fact becoming tiresome about health. Of course, everyone should do all they can to stay healthy. However, at some point the emphasis on cosmetic surgery seems to be motivated by a compelling fear that looking old is unnatural, when in fact it is the most natural thing in the world. Too much effort to deny the aging process not only is ultimately self-defeating but it leads to **ageism,** discrimination against old people.

Ageism in health care settings results in listening to older patients less carefully, treating them mechanically rather than with warmth, giving older people less time generally, or being patronizing. Being too busy to spend time with an older patient implies that the aged have lower social value. Like anyone being treated poorly, the aged pick up on this behavior. The message being communicated is that older people have less status and are less important as individuals.

Manifestations of ageism are also reflected in poor self-image among older people, which may contribute to a lack of self-esteem and perhaps depression. If being young and beautiful was all that brought meaning to an individual's life, then that person is going to have a tough time later in life. All of the exercise and face-lifting in the world ultimately will be a failure. It is not uncommon to find a kind of self-hatred among some aging people, although most people in late life are high in life satisfaction (Figure 1-5).

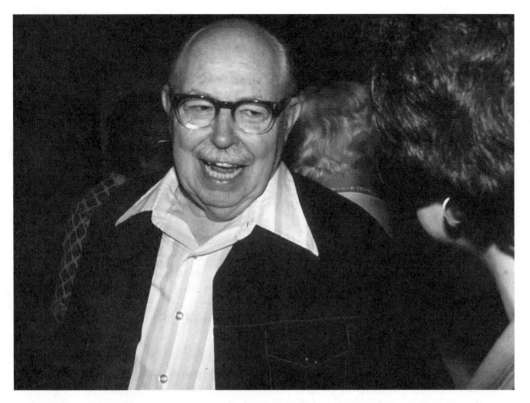

Figure 1-5 *Most older people are high in life satisfaction.*

HETEROGENEITY AMONG THE AGED

A universally accepted finding of gerontological research is that people become more heterogeneous over time, which often comes as a surprise to those who have given little thought to aging or who have little experience with older people. For those who have associated only with the young and remained segregated from the old, it is common to assume that all older people are alike in many ways, that they are homogeneous.

A common first assignment in introductory gerontology classes is for students to interview three older people. Many students interview their own grandparents. Typical remarks like these are recorded: "I never really talked with my grandfather before." "My grandmother had some really neat experiences." "We wound up talking for four hours—it was great!" Another prevailing theme found is the great number of differences that students find among the older people they have interviewed. Older people can be like living history books—each with a very different story.

COMMUNICATING WITH OLDER PEOPLE

There are several approaches that can be used to improve communication when working with older adults in health care environments.

Using Simple Language.   Older people can be intimidated in health care settings, especially those who have had little experience with doctors and hospitals. Health care professionals may be perceived to be powerful in a high-tech world. Professionals who use language that is difficult or impossible for laypersons to understand may frighten the elderly. This situation is unfortunate in that the information presented by the health care professional might be vital for the elderly person when exploring treatment options. The goal of good communication should be to use plain and simple language so that the message is clear.

Older People Are Customers.   It is too easy to forget that the reason health care professionals have jobs is that people pay for their services. True, much of the actual payment in health care settings comes from insurance companies or Medicare. But, it should be realized that the individual who is entitled to those insurance or Medicare benefits has a choice. If health care consumers are treated inappropriately, they might not choose the same services again.

Sharing Control.   Professionals in health settings have a great deal to do with determining patients' health care **locus of control** (Goldsteen, Counte, and Goldsteen, 1994). *Locus* means "location." An individual's center of control can be either internal or external or somewhere in between. Those who are internally controlled are independent and take care of themselves. Externally controlled persons are dependent and look to others for care. Too often, professionals in health care settings impose decisions on their patients that are not especially welcome. Gerontological research indicates that older people who have an internal locus of control are much higher in life satisfaction (Palmore and Luikart, 1972). Those who have control taken away from them do not do well in terms of recovery. This can be manifested in fairly subtle ways, but the end result is that older people who get shoved around do not recover as well. In fact, many of them do not recover at all.

The wise health care professional reinforces patients' internal control by letting them make decisions and indicate their needs and desires. This practice is especially important with the elderly, who may be intimidated by the health care environment, by the institutional setting, and by all the people who seem to be busy and important. Special care should be taken with older individuals, asking them what they want and presenting choices to them in such clear terms that there can be no confusion about the alternatives.

This concept goes beyond meal and television program choices. It has been found that the reluctance among older people to give advance directives for life-sustaining interventions revolves around their lack of understanding about just what these treatments mean (Luptak and Boult, 1994). Under the Patient Self-Determination Act of 1991, all people entering health care institutions and programs must be given the option of preparing a living will or designating someone to have durable power of attorney for health care. Some older patients, when given these choices in a perfunctory manner, simply check off that they want all life-sustaining means available used in their case. When the implications of this decision are explained, however, they often say, "Well, no, I don't want to live on a ventilator if there's no real chance of ever getting off of it." The professional who takes the time to explain things is in essence helping to empower older patients to make their own decisions. This consideration does not necessarily have to be just in major decision-making areas. Simply asking, "Would you like your breathing treatment before or after breakfast?" gives the individual some sense of control.

CASE STUDY

Admiral Peck, who had been in charge of things for much of his career, did not adapt well to a loss of control in retirement, and he had a stroke. At the nursing home, he was not able to articulate his needs, but he certainly could be ornery. Lennie, the orderly, did not like the admiral at all. He made it his task to make the old man's life miserable. He could also humiliate the old man. Powerless, the admiral turned his face to the wall and died.

1. What kinds of choices could Lennie have given the admiral that would have made him feel still in control?
2. What could other staff members have done to reinforce the admiral's perception of internal control?

Sensory Impairments. A substantial number of older people are blind (Figure 1-6), and many of those who can see need assistance. Failing eyesight or hearing can often be compensated for. If the patient has a hearing aid, make sure he is wearing it when you are talking to him, and make sure it is turned on. Speak slowly and clearly (but not loudly) to people, facing them so they can see your face when you are talking. Make sure they are wearing their glasses and that the glasses are clean. Be certain that there is plenty of light. Older people have difficulty adjusting to changes from bright environments to darker ones. When talking to older patients, try not to be standing with your back to the light. Eliminate distractions such as blaring televisions or radios. Establish presence by being on the same eye level. Do not be afraid to touch. With blind people, be sure to establish your presence verbally prior to touching them. If there is any question as to whether or not you have been understood, verify the message by asking the individual to repeat his or her understanding of what you have said. This provides an opportunity to clarify and eliminate misunderstandings. Take your time. It is hard to empower people who do not understand you.

Taking Time with Patients. Because older people often have sensory impairments, and many have cognitive impairments as well, dealing with them effectively often takes time. It is important to identify yourself and explain all procedures you are going to perform. Many older people resent being called by their first name unless they have given permission. Something as simple as, "Mr. Jones, it's Mary from Respiratory Therapy; I'm here to help you with your breathing treatment," sets the stage, orients the patient, eliminates the possibility of surprise, and is simple good manners.

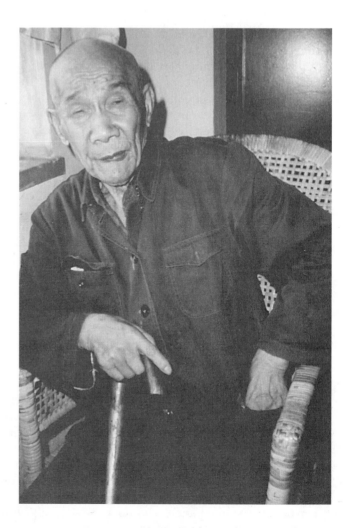

Figure 1-6 *The majority of blind people are older people.*

People pick up on the cues if you are too busy to stop and chat, give some comfort, or ask or answer a question. If a person needs to talk, sit down and let her talk. If this is impossible, make an appointment. Tell her you cannot talk right this minute, but that you will be back, and specify the exact time when you will be back. Handle this appointment exactly the way you would handle any important appointment—that is, be on time.

If time is limited, sit down and say, "I've only got five minutes, but right now they're your five minutes." This gives older individuals an immediate indication of a schedule, so they can get right down to what they need to share. Taking time with people lets them know that you think what they have to say is important. Often you will learn successful approaches with particular patients by taking time to know them.

Encouraging Reminiscence.   The life review is described in greater detail in the next chapter. For now, what is important is to realize that older people have a history and that they need to share it. It is the wise therapist who takes time to learn from patients. Listening to life stories is an especially effective way of establishing rapport. Patients are more likely to listen to what you have to say if they perceive they can trust you. Much of this trust can be built up over time by listening to the life stories that older people may be willing to share. Trust can be vital to compliance with a therapy plan. If patients trust the therapist, they will be more likely to listen and follow directions.

Sharing Feelings.   The foundation of a sympathetic understanding of others is based on letting them know you have an appreciation of what they are going through. It is inappropriate to claim **empathy**—knowledge based on having the same experience—unless you have had the same experience. Instead of saying, "I know just how you feel," you could say, "I can imagine how this feels."

SUMMARY

Gerontology and geriatrics are multidisciplinary; many professions contribute expertise in the care of the aged. Aging is a process, not an event, and people often seem to age at different rates, as do organs and systems. Social, psychological, and physical aspects of aging are often closely interrelated.

The aging population is growing faster than any other segment of society; the oldest old population is increasing the fastest. Because fewer young people die of communicable diseases, there has been an expansion of the population living into later life. As more people enter later life, there are more people presenting with the diseases of later life, and most of these diseases are chronic. The number of older, chronically ill people will dramatically increase in the twenty-first century when the postwar baby boomers become senior citizens.

Maximum life span will probably not be extended in the foreseeable future. The implication of the rectangularization of the survival curve is that more people will continue to live through childhood and midlife; they will live long enough to get old. Thus, there is a continuing likelihood of further extension of *average* life expectancy with new medical discoveries and better treatment modalities for middle-aged and older patients. The emergence of universal chronic illness is already being experienced, and most health care practitioners can anticipate taking care of many older, chronically ill people.

There are many ways to maintain rapport with older people. The most important is allowing people to maintain control over their lives and make decisions for themselves.

Review Questions

1. Why would older people as a group have a greater need for respiratory care than younger individuals?

2. What is the difference between gerontology and geriatrics?
3. What professional disciplines contribute to geriatrics?
4. What changes might we anticipate in our culture as the population ages?
5. What are the causes underlying the rectangularization of the survival curve?
6. Describe some of the implications of extension of the life span.
7. In what ways can we contribute to people maintaining internal control?

References

Fries, J. F., and Crapo, L. M. (1981). *Vitality and aging: Implications of the rectangular curve.* San Francisco: Freeman.

Goldsteen, R. L., Counte, M. A., and Goldsteen, K. (1994). Examining the relationship between health locus of control and the use of medical care services. *Journal of Aging and Health, 6,* 314–335.

Luptak, M. K., and Boult, C. (1994). A method for increasing elders' use of advance directives. *The Gerontologist, 34,* 409–412.

Minkler, M., and Robertson, A. (1991). The ideology of "age/race wars": Deconstructing a social problem. *Ageing and Society, 11,* 1–11.

National Center for Health Statistics (1996, October 4). *Monthly Vital Statistics Report, 45* (3). Hyattsville, MD: U.S. Public Health Service.

Palmore, E. B., and Luikart, C. (1972). Health and social factors related to life satisfaction. *Journal of Health and Social Behavior, 13,* 68–80.

Thorson, J. A. (1995). *Aging in a changing society.* Belmont, CA: Wadsworth.

CHAPTER TWO

PSYCHOSOCIAL ISSUES

activity theory
affective disorders
age normative
Alzheimer's disease
anomie
bipolar disorder
centenarians

confidant
continuity theory
disengagement theory
exchange theory
filial obligation
life review

longitudinal research
manic
multi-infarct dementia
organic disorders
paranoid
paraphrenia

LEARNING OBJECTIVES

After completing this chapter, the reader should be able to:

1. Enumerate ways that old people confront social loss.
2. Describe the concept of personality continuity over time.
3. Differentiate the activity, disengagement, and exchange theories of aging.
4. Describe how a confidant acts as a buffer against the forces of isolation.
5. Define stress inoculation and stress overload.
6. Explain the relationship of sick role behavior, external locus of control, and helplessness.
7. Explain the importance of the life review process.
8. List several cognitive disorders seen more frequently in later life.

INTRODUCTION

Much of this text deals with the physiological aspects of geriatric respiratory therapy and with the physiology of the aging process itself. It is also necessary to look more closely at social and psychological issues in gerontology in order to have a better understanding of older persons.

This chapter examines perceptions of aging as a part of the social world of the elderly. It also discusses other elements important to social gerontology, including aging people and their social networks, relationships, and role transitions. The chapter explores psychological development across the life span, with a special focus on psychological problems more common in later life. Implications for the respiratory care practitioner in dealing with older adults are emphasized.

SOCIAL ASPECTS OF GERONTOLOGY

What is it like to be old? What is it like to see life as increasingly limited? It may be difficult for a younger person to take on the perspective of measuring life as the accumulation of many years plus relatively few remaining years. Through most of youth and young adulthood people see the future as an almost infinite highway. In late life, the perspective changes. Life is mostly history. This change in point of view occurs gradually. However, it is inevitable for all who become old.

INDIVIDUAL DIFFERENCES

People not only age at different rates but in different ways. For some, the realization of advancing years may be seen as a triumph, as an accumulation of accomplishments and satisfaction. At the other extreme are those whose lives deteriorate into nothingness. For most older people, the prospect of gaining maturity is seen as positive, but weighed against it is the accommodation of a narrowing social world. Added to this situation is a realization of aging as a social process of adaptation to loss.

Loss of physical vitality is a fact of life for most, especially the very old. Loss of friends and loved ones is a fact of life as well. Socially, gerontologists speak of role loss as important to older people, and loss of status and self-esteem are also important. Despite these multiple losses, old age is not always perceived as negative. Many older people are living happy, productive lives, high in life satisfaction, often with the support of friends and family (Figure 2-1).

ADULT SOCIALIZATION

At an earlier time in the study of social gerontology, much was made of the concept of **anomie** or normlessness among the aged. Gerontologists questioned whether or not older people were particularly concerned with who they were, or who they were to be. The the-

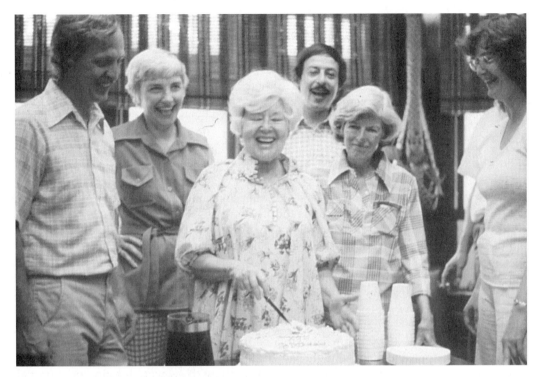

Figure 2-1 *Friends and family contribute to satisfaction in later life.*

ory was that older people had to confront many losses, including the loss of job through retirement, the resultant loss of social status due to loss of employment, the loss of physical integrity associated with the processes of biological aging, and the accumulation of the effects of trauma and disease over time. There was also the loss of strength and physical beauty, the loss of companionship due to retirement and widowhood, the sensory losses over the course of years, and the loss of sexuality associated with physical and social losses. Compounding these losses was the loss of norms. Old people were said to have few examples to follow in terms of being socialized into later life. Thus, old age appeared to be something of a wasteland. Old people had no real role in society.

With the growth of social gerontology as an area of study over recent years, however, there has been an increasing amount of research indicating that normlessness is not a major problem for most older people. Loneliness may well be a problem for many, but a lack of identity seems to not be an important issue. This is probably because of personality continuity across the life span. Basically, people remain pretty much the same over time. Those who have developed ego integrity in adulthood carry it into later life. In fact, for most people, old age is not seen as a separate stage in life as much as it is a continuation of adulthood.

Attitudes Toward Aging.   Individuals are, nevertheless, socialized into old age. Socialization is the process by which people learn society's rules. An understanding of age-appropriate behavior might be an example of this socialization. At early stages in life, children are told to grow up or to act their age. At the other end of life, acting one's age may have an entirely different meaning. That is, there are things that society sees as inappropriate for older people to do. Common expressions such as "There's no fool like an old fool" exemplify this concept. There are social pressures to conform to what others expect. There are certain attitudes that are held by most people, and these societal attitudes make up a system of norms to which older people—and the rest of us—are expected to adhere.

Attitudes socialize people into later life. In some cases, these social forces can be codified formally as folkways, norms, mores, or laws. Whatever they are called, they tend to powerfully reinforce what people in a society can and cannot do. If these norms are violated, society may take sanctions against the violator.

Think, for example, of an instance of age-inappropriate behavior. Say that an 88-year-old decides to go bungee jumping. A sense of reckless adventure is seen as all right for a young person, but certainly not for an old one. Say that the same 88-year-old decides to wed a spouse of 26. This might be a violation of age norms that really causes tongues to wag. Just as a 12-year-old can no longer pitch a tantrum that might have been tolerated in a 6-year-old, someone who is nearing 90 can no longer do things thought to be more appropriate for a teenager.

On the other hand, if age norms are violated in minor matters, society's response may be a chuckle of approval. People might say "right on" to the old woman who rides a motorcycle or the old man who takes up mountain climbing. However, this kind of approval could also be seen as patronizing in some ways. It represents a kind of ageism in that the question is raised in the first place. It would be no one else's affair if a 30-year-old woman started riding a motorcycle. Why should the situation be any different for an 80-year-old? Events in life are seen as **age normative.**

Hagestad and Neugarten (1985) speak of a "social clock" that regulates our lives. There is a time to get married, a time to have children, a time to work, and a time to quit working. Although the parameters of these expectations of appropriate times and events may have expanded in recent years, they are still present.

Changing Norms.   Some of society's norms and expectations change. Divorce might be seen as a good illustration of how expectations of normative behavior evolve. When Adlai Stevenson ran for president in 1952, much was made of the fact that he had been divorced. This had become a nonissue by the time Ronald Reagan, who had also been divorced, was elected to the presidency in 1980. Racial attitudes might be another example of social change. Mixed-race marriages in the early 1900s were actually illegal in most U.S. states. Even after the laws were changed, marrying a person of another race was viewed by many with deep disapproval. Although this issue may still be controversial for some, it represents an example of norms in evolution. What society sees as acceptable changes over time.

Many older people are constantly adapting to new ways of seeing things. If they fail to keep up, they might be seen by others as old-fashioned or set in their ways. Social change puts the aged under constant pressure to adapt. They may lament these changes. It is common to hear older people complain about how things were different in past years, and there may be a sense of nostalgia for earlier, simpler times. Nevertheless, older people are well practiced at adaptation. They have had to do a lot of it over the course of their lives.

History-Normative Perspective. There are also history-normative events one might anticipate finding among the generation that is now old. Older people born prior to 1930 have all lived through the Great Depression and World War II. The oldest old may also remember Prohibition and World War I. Values that they learned as young people arising out of these events often persist.

An example of a history-normative characteristic common among many older people is thrift. Those who were children during the Depression and World War II remember scarcities that today's young people have never had to confront. For this reason, it may be that some older people have a difficult time throwing things out. They were raised with a "waste not, want not" philosophy. Since older people are constantly confronted by loss, it may be no wonder that some seek to hold on to material things. Thus, it is common for the aged to pack their residences too full of furniture and other material possessions. Two things are going on: They are trying to hold on to familiar things in the face of social loss, and they remember how difficult it once was in their lives to acquire those objects.

Role Transitions. Two of the important, expected changes that come with later life are retirement for those who have been employed and widowhood for those who have been married. Thus, there is an anticipated role transition for most of the older population. In actuality, most older people make transitions in several different roles, including from worker or producer to leisure participant, from spouse to widow or widower, from parent to grandparent or great-grandparent, and perhaps from an image of an active person to one having a more passive existence.

Theories of Social Gerontology. Several theories of social gerontology attempt to explain these role transitions (Thorson, 1995). One, for example, holds that those who maintain the highest level of activity in later life are the ones who adapt best to old age. This **activity theory** of aging says that the successful older person replaces lost roles and activities with new ones over time. The vital older person does not retire to a rocking chair, but seeks to become involved in a number of new things to fill his or her life with meaning. In a sense, this is like another theory of social gerontology, the **continuity theory,** which says that old age is really an extension of middle age. There is continuity of personality over time, and the person who was active in late middle age will probably be happiest remaining active in old age. Shy people will remain shy, and outgoing people will remain outgoing; there will be some replacement of activities, but the general thrust of life will be essentially similar.

By contrast, the **disengagement theory** of aging says that old age is more developmental. Later life is seen as a genuinely separate part of life with its own roles and norms. Just as people are seeking less active roles because of slowing physical processes, society is starting to replace them in the world of work and public affairs. Thus, disengagement is a mutual push-pull kind of process. People tend to become disengaged from active roles at the same time society finds less need for them (Figure 2-2). People who try to hang on to formerly important roles are bound to be disappointed when they are literally shoved into inactivity.

The disengagement theory may be seen as less optimistic than the activity theory of continuous involvement in meaningful roles. But no doubt the pattern of aging that is best varies greatly among individuals. Some genuinely are ready to put it on the shelf and enjoy sedentary activities. Others hope to wear out rather than rust out and will keep going as long as their strength holds up. Most people, of course, disengage from some roles gladly and seek to hold on to others. There is one additional theory of social gerontology that has almost universal application.

The **exchange theory** looks at interactions between and among individuals as a system of trade-offs. As an illustration, Stinnet and DeFrain (1985) examined long-term marriages to see what it was that kept people married for 40 or 50 years or longer. The almost universal response was mutual regard, but it was also important that each was making a contribution to the maintenance of the relationship. Further, each of the partners in long-term marriages felt that they were getting more of a reward out of the relationship than they put into it. This is a good example of exchange theory as it applies to later life: People seek to maintain those relationships that reward them the most, relative to their investment. Exchanges are not strictly on a calculated basis; love is also important.

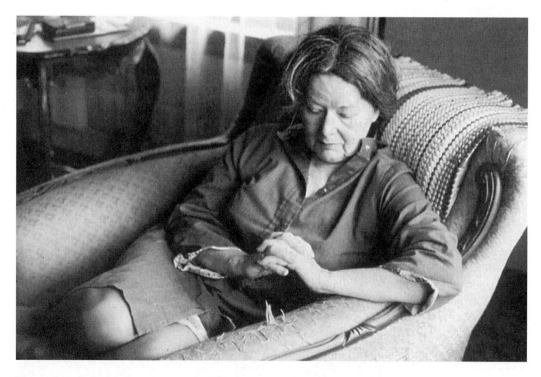

Figure 2-2 *Disengagement is seen as a legitimate role for many older people.*

In terms of older people and those around them, the exchange theory holds that a sense of **filial obligation** makes adult children continue to provide services for their aged parents. They seek no particular reward; they do something not because it is expected but because they want to. In other areas of life one might expect more of a mutuality of exchange. For example, older people certainly do things for each other.

IMPLICATIONS OF ADAPTATION TO LOSS

Many of the changes older people confront are in a negative direction. In particular, older people for the most part are no longer seen as being important in an ageist society. It is little wonder that many older people have problems with loss of self-esteem.

A practical implication for the practitioner dealing with older patients comes from a realization that they may be reluctant to try new things. This becomes a critical problem when, for example, technical aspects of self-care are being taught to a person who is being discharged home. Fear of failure is high, and many may be hesitant to attempt things that seem relatively simple to the therapist. Health care professionals have a teaching function that cannot be overemphasized in its importance. Patience, reassurance, and repeated positive reinforcement are critical. If older persons are to regain independence, they may need to learn things that seem exceedingly challenging. Remember that they have had it emphasized again and again that "you can't teach an old dog new tricks." However, unless there is cognitive impairment, even very old people can continue to be effective learners. A gradual approach with much repetition may be the key to teaching older patients techniques of self-monitoring and therapies they need to know either for their own care or for the care of their spouse. Once a skill has been taught, it may be necessary to verify a number of times that it is being done correctly. Practice brings rewards and bolsters self-confidence.

There is a second implication for the practitioner. Because of history-normative influences, older people may have a different understanding of what is proper. A sense of modesty, for example, may be both highly developed and fairly rigid among some older people. They are not used to—and do not like—having certain parts of their bodies uncovered. Therapists should be sensitive to this modesty. Also, in their earlier years, they did not address older individuals by their first names. A sign of respect was to use the last name, for example, "Mr. Jones," or, "Mrs. Smith." Certainly, they did not think it at all polite to call someone older than themselves by their first name or by a pet name such as "Honey" or "Sweetie." Health care professionals should be very conscious of simple good manners in this regard. When in doubt, it is best to ask people how they wish to be addressed.

As older people are constantly in the situation of having to adapt to loss, there is no reason for the therapist to make this worse. Becoming impatient or short with older individuals only makes them less confident and less able to maintain their independence. Treating them as if they cannot learn will only reinforce negative self-images. Using patronizing terms or names, or talking about people in their presence as if they were not there, robs people of their dignity and individuality. Older people have enough losses to adapt to without having to confront the additional burden of disrespect. One of the best things the respiratory care practitioner can seek to do in interventions with the aged is prevent loss of autonomy.

SOCIAL IMPLICATIONS OF HOME CARE

The family may be critical to the success of the therapy because of increasing emphasis on outpatient or home care. Many of the therapies formerly delivered in the hospital are now performed in the home. It may not be reasonable to expect that the older patient himself will be able to take on all of the care responsibilities, and a caregiver—usually a family member—may become the one who performs some or all of the therapy. Delivery of care by professionals visiting the patient's residence may or may not be entirely possible. Often, it is the case that a primary caregiver who lives with or near the older patient becomes in effect a service extender. The therapist sets up a program and carries out the critical duties, while a family member may be responsible for carrying out instructions and monitoring the patient. Thus, the presence of a family member becomes critical to maintaining the independence of the older adult. The availability of a partner varies widely by age and gender (Table 2-1).

TABLE 2-1   Marital Status by Age and Sex, Percentages, 1994

Age and Sex	Single	Married	Widowed	Divorced
Male				
18 to 19 years old	96.9	2.9	—	0.2
20 to 24 years old	81.0	17.9	0.1	1.0
25 to 29 years old	48.4	47.0	0.1	4.5
30 to 34 years old	30.1	62.4	0.1	7.4
35 to 39 years old	19.7	68.8	0.3	11.2
40 to 44 years old	10.8	76.3	0.5	12.3
45 to 54 years old	6.9	80.5	1.0	11.6
55 to 64 years old	6.6	80.9	3.7	8.9
65 to 74 years old	4.8	80.1	9.4	5.6
75 years old and older	3.8	71.0	22.6	2.6
Female				
18 to 19 years old	90.0	9.6	—	0.4
20 to 24 years old	66.8	31.0	0.1	2.2
25 to 29 years old	33.1	58.6	0.3	8.0
30 to 34 years old	19.3	69.5	0.5	10.7
35 to 39 years old	12.5	73.8	1.1	12.6
40 to 44 years old	9.1	73.8	1.9	15.3
45 to 54 years old	5.4	73.4	4.4	16.7
55 to 64 years old	4.2	69.1	14.4	12.2
65 to 74 years old	3.7	54.0	35.2	7.1
75 years old and older	5.4	26.6	63.8	4.2

Source: *U.S. Bureau of the Census. Statistical Abstract of the United States, 114th ed., 1995.*

There is a wide discrepancy between the genders in the proportions that are married and widowed. Over 70 percent of men age 75 and older have a surviving spouse; this is not the case for women. Only a little more than a quarter of women in that age category have a living husband. The percentage of widows begins to increase sharply after age 55. Thus, a spousal caregiver is much more likely to be present if the patient is male. For female patients, it may be more likely that the family caregiver is an adult child.

Some older people, however, are genuinely isolated, and they tend to be the ones most vulnerable to institutionalization. If an in-home caregiver is not available, then the individual needing care has to get it somewhere else. Those without family resources are at about twice the risk of institutionalization. A little over 10 percent of the elderly are isolates. Isolated older people not only have higher rates of institutionalization but they also have much higher mortality rates (Steinbach, 1992).

The majority, though, do have families, and most older people remain intimately involved with their families. (Figure 2-3). One recent study of a random sample of 500 adults in their seventies and eighties found their mean number of visits from family members was 2.37 per week. Only 30 percent had not received a visit from a family member during the week prior to the interview, and only 14 percent had not received a phone call from a family member (Thorson, 1995).

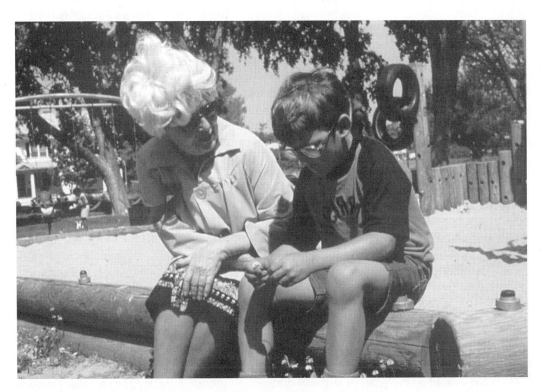

Figure 2-3 *Most older people remain intimately involved with their families.*

Among the oldest old, those 85 and above, the situation deteriorates. Almost all in one study were widowed or lived alone with no surviving child living nearby. There is a risk among the oldest old of outliving their families. According to Johnson and Troll (1992), about one-third had a family member who served as a caregiver and another 35 percent said they had one available if needed. The remaining 29 percent had no family member who would be available in times of need. While nursing home placement rates for the 65 and older population taken as a whole generally run about 4 to 5 percent, among those age 85 and above the rate of institutionalization is about 22 percent for males and almost 30 percent for females. The higher rate for women is explained by the fact that they are much less likely to have a surviving spousal caregiver.

Physical caretaking, of course, is not the only function of family. There are social and psychological benefits to those who interact with significant others. Grandchildren, in particular, give older individuals a sense of satisfaction. It is especially important for some to see family continuity stretching into future generations.

Social Networks and Confidants.   Family members, especially siblings and adult children, provide a pool of confidants for older individuals who are in danger of becoming isolated. A **confidant** is a person in whom one may confide, a trusted significant other who values the relationship enough to take the time to listen to an older person's deepest thoughts and feelings. Whereas many friendships are at fairly superficial levels, a confidant relationship, by contrast, represents a particularly strong bond. Men's confidants tend to be their wives, and if they become widowed, there is a very good chance that men will become isolated. This may in part explain the extraordinarily high suicide rate among older white males, a topic we discuss in Chapter 8. In fact, older men who lose a spouse are twice as likely to die of any cause than men who remain coupled (Steinbach, 1992).

This is not the case, however, among older widowed women. They have the same mortality odds as other women in the same age group who have not experienced the death of a spouse. This situation is explained by the greater likelihood of older women to maintain an intact social network, often having several people in whom to confide. Social networks for most older women go well beyond the bounds of family.

PSYCHOLOGICAL ISSUES

Several issues related to adult development in later life are introduced early in this chapter. With the continuity theory, for example, it can be seen that the self remains fairly constant over time. People's views of the world often have been shaped by history-normative events. This life perspective is unlikely to change with the onset of old age. Further, most older people successfully adapt to change, even change that is in a negative direction. The importance of the maintenance of a social network to the psychological health of older people is an example of the multidisciplinary nature of gerontology.

There are a number of issues that should be explored further. Do older people really have a more difficult time learning things? Is cognitive impairment more common late in life? What should be expected in terms of diminished mental capacity? These issues are discussed next, as well as a number of psychological processes important to older adults.

STRESS AND ADAPTATION

Despite the general concept that older people adapt to change pretty successfully, there are major life events that precipitate psychological and physical problems. Not all are perceived the same way by all older people. Widowhood, for example, seems to have a greater impact on males than females. Perhaps this is because it is more common for older women to lose their husbands, and therefore they may have some sense of expectation. The stress of loss is still there, and coping with being alone and accomplishing grief work is still necessary, but the loss may be less shocking for women. Similarly, people who are working can see retirement coming for a long time. Loss of a career can be stressful, but at least it can be anticipated. Retirement, too, has positive as well as negative consequences.

Stress and Life Change. In theory, foreseen changes and losses might have less impact than unexpected ones. There is more time to prepare and think through eventualities associated with an anticipated stressful event. In 1967, Holmes and Rahe sought a way to quantify the stress associated with life change. Their Social Readjustment Rating Scale lists forty-three different stress-producing events, from minor violations of the law at the low end of the scale to death of a spouse at the other extreme. Other high-stress events include divorce, marital separation, jail term, death of a close family member, and personal injury or illness. What was unique about the Holmes–Rahe scale was that numerical values were assigned to individual events. Some years later, Thorson and Thorson (1981) pointed out that at least sixteen of these events were much more likely to happen in the lives of older adults (Table 2-2).

The idea underlying the Holmes–Rahe scale is that stress is cumulative, and that ultimately one more straw will break the camel's back. Various studies since its publication have shown that people with too many stressful events in their lives in a short period of time indeed are more likely to get sick, have psychological problems, or even die. This situation leads to the concept of stress overload, as well as an underlying principle of stress management.

Older people adjusting to major changes, such as retirement or death of a spouse, are well advised to wait some time before making additional changes. A recently widowed person, for example, should wait six months to a year before selling his or her home and moving to a retirement community. The change in location right after bereavement might add additional, unnecessary stress.

In a subsequent article (Thorson and Thorson, 1986), it was pointed out that in some ways the Holmes–Rahe scale is not all that appropriate for counseling older adults. Although the underlying principle of stress overload leading to physical or psychological trauma is valid, there are additional things going on in the lives of older adults that make this general scale less useful.

People who have good coping skills may handle the stress associated with change better than others. It has been shown, for example, that older people seem to cope better than younger adults with natural disasters (Bell, Kara, and Batterson, 1978). Perhaps older people simply have more experience in putting life change into perspective. Also, the Holmes–Rahe scale might not be appropriate because of the unique social situation of older people. Something not on the scale, the death of a grandchild, for example, might be perceived by an older person as much more stressful than the death of a spouse.

TABLE 2-2   **Stressful Events More Likely to Occur in Later Life**

Life Event	Point Value
Death of spouse	100
Death of close family member	63
Personal injury or illness	53
Retirement	45
Change in health of family member	44
Sex difficulties	39
Change in financial state	38
Death of a close friend	37
Change in number of arguments with spouse	35
Son or daughter leaving home	29
Change in living conditions	25
Revision of personal habits	24
Change in residence	20
Change in recreation	19
Change in social activities	18
Change in sleeping habits	16

Source: *Adapted from T. H. Holmes and R. H. Rahe (1967). The social readjustment rating scale.* Journal of Psychosomatic Research, 11, *213–218.*

Institutionalization is not on the Holmes–Rahe scale, yet it is a significant fear of older adults. Going to a nursing home implies a loss of freedom of choice. This loss of independence might be seen as disastrous by some older people. This issue leads to a discussion of control. Recall that in Chapter 1 it was mentioned that it is important to let older people make choices, to let them have some semblance of control over their lives.

Loss of this personal control often happens in health care institutions. Research has shown, for example, that those who are relocated against their will have an especially high mortality rate. They may react to a combination of perceived stresses with a helplessness response, something that the nursing literature refers to as sick role behavior (Thorson, 1988). These patients often fail to thrive and many give up the will to live (Seligman, 1975). The stress of the loss of personal control associated with an involuntary relocation is seen as a disaster by many older people. Expectation in this instance may be a predictor of behavior. Perhaps people placed in nursing homes feel that they are supposed to die.

Coping Mechanisms.   Why do some people give up the ghost, seemingly without a struggle, and others persist in the face of crushing burdens? Perhaps the answer can be found in the way they have approached other problems earlier in life, in their personal adaptive mechanisms.

It has been found that personality is basic to the individual, that it does not change very much over time. In the study of human development, personality in adulthood is thought of as pretty much a constant. Certainly, people learn new things over the course of their lives; they integrate concepts and often try new ways of dealing with things. Their essential personality makeup, however, remains much the same. Consider meeting a friend at a class reunion after being separated for 30 or 40 years. The characteristics that made this individual a friend will most likely still be present.

People do not change so much as they react to events. Persons constantly faced with adversity may draw inward or become angry. Others faced with problems may react expansively and generously. The ways they go about facing life's problems are probably fairly typical across the course of adult life.

Personality is made up of a number of traits; theorists differ as to exactly how many and what traits are present, but all agree that there are certain basic elements of personality. Being outgoing is an example of a trait. Introverts who are not naturally outgoing will have to make a concerted effort if they wish to act a different way, whereas some people are just natural extroverts.

Contrasted to traits are states, which are reactions to social situations in which people find themselves. Anger might be seen as a state. Everyone gets angry, but most people get over it. Anger is a temporary state, not a constant personality trait. If a person consistently reacts to situations with hostility and aggression, though, this might be a part of her basic personality structure. This characteristic might then be seen as a trait.

Added to this basic foundation of traits, the tools of personality are found in the adaptive mechanisms, which change over time, as people grow and develop throughout life. One system of adaptive mechanisms is explained by psychiatrist George Vaillant (1977) in his study of a sample that has been followed since 1938 (Table 2-3). These subjects began as 19- and 20-year-olds and are now in their eighties. This kind of **longitudinal research** is important so that changes that take place in the same individuals over time can be observed. Vaillant says that people have a characteristic clustering of adaptive mechanisms that they typically use to confront problems. This cluster of coping mechanisms can be at a fairly low, immature level, or it can be at a higher level achieved through maturation.

It is expected that people will achieve the mature mechanisms as they progress through adulthood. If they are adapting successfully, they will have left the earlier mechanisms behind in childhood. Only those who are mentally ill will characteristically use the coping mechanisms found at the lowest levels. Most adults, especially older adults, will consistently have a grouping of Level III and especially Level IV mechanisms. These adaptive mechanisms have been gained through development and growth of the personality throughout adulthood.

Implications of Stress and Adaptation. It is possible in later life, particularly if cognitive impairment is present, for some people to slip back in the level of their adaptive mechanisms. This circumstance may be particularly true of the frail elderly who are confronted with numerous problems and losses. For example, the patient who might in better times react to life changes with suppression or anticipation may instead react to a crisis with repression and hypochondriasis.

Life is like a motion picture, with a beginning, middle, and end. Often, when caring for geriatric clients, the only thing seen by health care professionals is a snapshot. In order to

---

TABLE 2-3   Vaillant's Categorization of Adaptive Mechanisms

Level I: Psychotic Mechanisms
   1. Delusional projection: Frank delusions about external reality, generally involving thoughts of persecution.
   2. Denial: Denial of external reality.
   3. Distortion: Grossly reshaping external reality to suit inner needs.

Level II: Immature Mechanisms
   4. Projection: Attributing one's own unacknowledged feelings to others.
   5. Schizoid fantasy: Use of fantasy, avoidance of intimacy, and the use of eccentricity to repel others.
   6. Hypochondriasis: Complaints of pain or illness, wishes to be dependent.
   7. Passive-aggressive behavior: Aggression toward others expressed indirectly through passivity or directed against the self.
   8. Acting out: Delinquent or impulsive acts and "tempers."

Level III: Neurotic Defenses
   9. Intellectualization: Isolation, rationalization, ritual, magical thinking, and busy-work. The idea is in the consciousness, but the affect is missing.
   10. Repression: Inexplicable naivete or forgetting, failure to acknowledge input. The feeling is in consciousness, but the idea is missing.
   11. Displacement: Redirection of feelings, wit with hostile intent, phobias, and prejudices.
   12. Reaction formation: Behavior diametrically opposed to an unacceptable impulse; "hating" someone one really likes.
   13. Dissociation: Hysterical conversion reactions, short-term refusal to perceive responsibility for one's acts or feelings.

Level IV: Mature Mechanisms
   14. Altruism: Constructive service to others, generosity.
   15. Humor: Like hope, humor permits one to focus on reality and deal with what is too terrible to be borne.
   16. Suppression: Conscious decision to postpone dealing with an impulse or conflict; keeping a stiff upper lip.
   17. Anticipation: Realistic planning for the future, especially future discomfort.
   18. Sublimation: Indirect expression of instincts without adverse consequences; instincts are channeled rather than dammed or diverted; successful artistic expression is a classic example of sublimation.

Source: *Adapted from George E. Vaillant (1977).* Adaptation to life. *Boston: Little, Brown.*

---

have an appreciation for what the individual is really like, it is necessary to talk to family members. The use of immature defenses such as schizoid fantasy or passive-aggressive behavior may or may not be characteristic of the individual. Relapse to use of less mature mechanisms may be only temporary.

Practitioners need to work with people where they are, not where they are "supposed" to be. It is too easy to form value judgments, to like or dislike patients because of their behavior. The professional should not draw hasty conclusions and deem someone as "good" or "bad." It may take considerable maturity on the practitioner's part to reserve judgment and deal with people as they are, even in their worst moments.

On the other hand, the practitioner should not be taken aback by the older person who uses the most mature of the adaptive mechanisms. People who characteristically use humor and anticipation, for example, may speak matter-of-factly about their impending death. Many older people have planned their own funerals and are able to talk candidly—even joke—about the end of life. Others responding with the mature mechanisms approach the termination of life with suppression, and many use altruism; they are interested in doing good for those who will follow after them. Respiratory care practitioners, especially very young ones, may have a difficult time dealing with such candor. Too often, people want to rush in and assure dying patients that they in fact will live for many more years. This may be because the fledgling practitioner has yet to work out her own feelings about death. Older people do not need to be lied to about their prognosis. If they want to talk about the end of life, their needs should not be denied.

THE LIFE REVIEW

Assessing life as it comes to a close is a normal psychological process that happens to almost everyone. The **life review** is an ongoing process, rather than an event, and it is brought on by the realization of impending death (Butler, 1963). This does not necessarily mean that people who reflect back upon the meaning of life are terminally ill. Rather, this process takes place when the individual realizes that the remainder of life is limited. The life review can occur among people in their sixties who are perfectly healthy. They see that their contemporaries are starting to die, and they seek to mentally take stock of who they are and where they have been, which may well be for the purpose of planning where they are going. Many people take on new interests, travels, or learning projects as a result of a life review.

The life review is a process of reminiscence where past events are spontaneously brought into the consciousness. Most people conclude from this process that they have led pretty good lives, all things considered. But a small percentage may become depressed or even suicidal, especially if they conclude that they have wasted their lives.

This reviewing of past events helps older people put life into perspective. Some may need to bend reality a little to find real self-acceptance. However, the process itself is usually a growth experience and one whereby older people acquire wisdom. People may realize, for example, that the true meaning of life is found not in the acquisition of material goods but in their relationships with others. Research has demonstrated that people who have accomplished a life review have much less death anxiety (Thorson and Powell, 1990). Perhaps they feel that much of their life's work has been accomplished. Others may feel that they have many things left to do, and some seem to buckle down to get it done. People often feel that goals that have been postponed must either be accomplished or, as often happens, revised.

Implications of the Life Review.   Some may feel that they need to make peace with others before it is too late. Here is another area where there is an important implication for the respiratory care practitioner. Health care professionals who deal with older people may be selected to share confidences and provide reassurance. It is not unprofessional to become somewhat involved in the lives of one's patients. For example, it may be necessary to call a patient's brother in another state and say that Mr. Jones regrets the feud the family has engaged in all these years and he wants to apologize for his bad behavior.

Becoming closely involved with the details of a patient's life will not happen often, of course, but it should not come as a surprise. At the very least, a common and normal outcome of the life review process is the need to share stories with other people. This may be an exercise in self-justification or merely a means by which people are able to put things into perspective. In either event, it is incumbent upon practitioners as professionals to sit still and listen. On a personal basis, when one's own older relatives wish to reminisce, it is a good thing to listen as well. The successful accomplishment of the life review process frequently involves active listening (Figure 2-4).

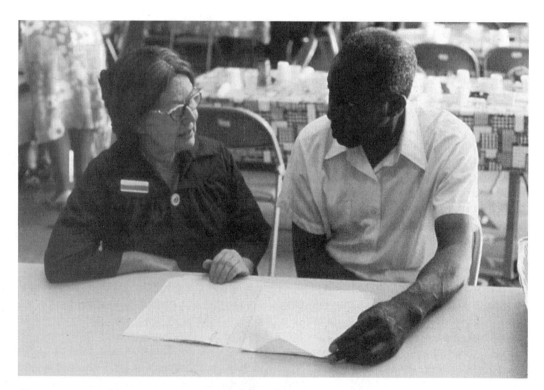

Figure 2-4   *Attentive listening helps individuals accomplish the life review process.*

COGNITION

No area of the psychology of aging is so clouded by stereotype and myth as is the assessment of cognitive abilities of older adults. Older persons themselves often buy into cultural biases and feel that they are slipping or slowing down in their mental processes. Memory lapses are commonly attributed to old age. Cognition, which usually is thought of as both learning and memory, seemingly is expected to decline by many people. Compounding the research in this area, it has been shown that many older adults have a higher fear of failure and appear to be less motivated in testing situations. Perhaps poorer results when comparing achievement test scores of the elderly with younger subjects might be explained to a certain degree by a lack of skill in test-taking strategies. Clerical skills are important in many paper-and-pencil tests. Those with slowing responses and perceptual difficulties naturally do not do well on timed tests. Sorting out what areas of intellect have genuine decline and what can be attributed to testing problems can be methodologically difficult.

There can be little doubt that samples of older people generally perform poorly in tests of mental abilities when compared with younger adults. It used to be thought that this evidence could be used to prove an overall theory of cognitive decline with chronological age. This made some sense: As strength and bodily integrity usually decline at a fairly predictable rate, so should mental abilities. Recent research, however, shows that the issue is much more complex (Thorson, 1995).

Learning, an important part of cognition, is dependent on two things: the senses and an intact cognitive structure in the brain. If the senses are impaired, if the person is deaf or has difficulty seeing, then less information is acquired. If the processing mechanism, the cognitive structure of the brain, is impaired, then less information is going to be processed. These are critical issues, as many older people have sensory impairments, which means that input is limited. In later life, the cognitive structure may also be impaired.

Intelligence is the ability to learn and remember. Many achievement tests that purport to measure intelligence do not in fact tap true mental abilities. Most of the research in learning and memory ignores practical and adaptive skills acquired through a lifetime of experience. Tests instead measure tasks that are much the same as those presented in academic settings. As might be expected, most older persons do poorly on these tests when compared with younger people. Few tests are able to adequately measure practical and adaptive skills. Here one might ask what intelligence really consists of: Is it the ability to memorize and repeat back a random list of words, or is it the ability to raise and nurture a large family on a limited budget? In other words, intelligence might mean different things to different people. Further, it is often difficult to sort out cognitive decline that is associated with disease from mental decline that may be characteristic of the aging process itself.

Most longitudinal studies of learning and memory among older samples show little in the way of measurable decline among the healthy elderly until at least the seventh decade of life (Thorson, 1995). This finding implies that many mental difficulties found in older populations probably are more the result of disease than of aging itself. Hypertension and small strokes that are the result of hypertension are often responsible for decreasing mental abilities in later life. There are other diseases as well that are more common in later life that may cause cognitive decline.

It may be helpful to describe exactly what is meant by cognitive decline. There can be little doubt that, given enough time, mental processes slow down. This can be seen best in samples of **centenarians,** people who have lived to be 100 years of age or older. One study of centenarians involved interviews with 166 men and women (Beard, 1968). Twenty percent of the interviewees could not say what they had eaten for their previous meal, over a quarter could not remember the president's name, and half could not remember the interviewer's name, all of which might be seen as short-term memory loss. Forty percent of the centenarians could not count forward five digits, and half of them could not count backward four digits, indicating problems with the basic cognitive structure of the brain. Only 54 percent in Beard's sample could follow a simple sequence of four or more steps. It was very clear that many of these people were demented and could not perform even simple mental tasks.

A more recent study of a sample of centenarians found pretty much the same thing: declines in intelligence and in both short- and long-term memory (Poon et al., 1992). It is important to note, however, that in this more recent study, problem-solving ability was tested as well. It had not declined appreciably—it was similar to the ability of a comparison sample of research subjects in their sixties.

Although it is clear that declining cognitive ability increases in very late life, it is also interesting to note that about half of these very old people did not have significant deficits. Some could still perform the tests they were given perfectly. Almost all could still carry on conversations and use language logically, which is a very complex mental task. Many had interesting things to say to the interviewers.

It is evident that some parts of the cognitive structure are more likely to remain intact. In general, abilities that are used seem to remain and those that are not used decline more rapidly. An implication of the research on cognitive abilities among the aged is that mental decline should not be seen as normal. Most often mental deterioration can be attributed to physical problems, usually disease. The kinds of mental problems commonly seen, such as confusion or forgetfulness, might be signs of reversible illness, not mental decline associated with old age itself. This leads to a more detailed discussion of mental problems more common in later life.

Dementia and Delirium.   The most prevalent mental problems in later life that affect cognition are dementia and delirium. Unfortunately, they are also the most frequently confused. True dementia is the result of a disease, such as **Alzheimer's,** or a physical process, such as **multi-infarct dementia,** which is caused by a series of small strokes. Delirium is a temporary condition that might be caused by overmedication, infection, hypothermia, alcohol poisoning, or congestive heart failure. Too often, people with delirium are misdiagnosed as being demented, as having an irreversible mental condition that cannot be treated. All other possible causes of disorganized behavior must be eliminated before arriving at a diagnosis of dementia.

Alzheimer's Disease.   Among the dementias, true Alzheimer's disease makes up at least half of all cases, with most of the remainder being accounted for by multi-infarct dementia, Parkinson's disease, brain tumor, and other neurological problems. There have been two analyses of major studies of the prevalence of Alzheimer's disease by age (Table 2-4).

TABLE 2-4   Two Analyses of Dementia of the Alzheimer's Type

Age Group	Analysis 1 (%)	Analysis 2 (%)
60–64 years	1.0	0.7
65–69 years	1.4	1.4
70–74 years	4.1	2.8
75–79 years	5.7	5.6
80–84 years	13.0	10.5
85–89 years	21.6	20.8
90–94 years	32.2	38.6

Source: *C. Brayne (1993). Research and Alzheimer's disease: An epidemiological perspective.* Psychological Medicine, 23, *287–296.*

The data in Table 2-4 indicate first that an assessment of the prevalence of Alzheimer's disease is imprecise; there is some discrepancy between the two analyses. However, these data also indicate that the condition is relatively rare among the young old and relatively common among the very old. About a third of people age 90 or older probably have some level of Alzheimer's disease. However, they probably will die of something else.

Alzheimer's disease is a progressive, dementing condition, characterized by gross mental deterioration. It is identified by neurofibrillary tangles found in the brain on autopsy. Presently, it is irreversible. People with Alzheimer's become progressively forgetful, have difficulty learning and remembering things, are confused and often irrational, and typically have some degree of personality change. The condition causes great distress among family members, and it often runs in families, which implies that its cause may be partly genetic. The person with Alzheimer's disease, however, often is not in any particular pain or great personal distress.

Multi-Infarct Dementia.   People with multi-infarct dementia are generally quite aware of their condition. They often are frustrated, as are most stroke victims, in that they have the words they want to say on the tip of their tongue, but they cannot express them. Like other stroke victims, there is some potential for the rehabilitation of those with multi-infarct dementia.

People who have had strokes are not always demented—it depends on which part of the brain has been affected by the stroke. They are seen by respiratory care practitioners more often than people with Alzheimer's disease because of common problems with swallowing or choking, which may lead to pneumonia.

Affective Disorders.   **Affective disorders** are differentiated from delirium and dementia, which are usually thought of as the **organic disorders** that influence cognition. Affective disorders typically have no organic cause, but are about equally common in later life as organic disorders—and can have an effect equally as devastating. Most prevalent among the affective disorders is depression.

Depression.   Depression is characterized by sleep disturbances, fatigue, and inactivity that is uncharacteristic of the individual. The person may wake up feeling tired, have gloomy or morbid thoughts, and have fatigue that is constant, that goes beyond tiredness after exertion. Lack of interest is another sign of depression. Kermis (1986) states that old age mimics depression. However, there are some things that clearly differentiate depression from moods that occur now and again among all older people: "Although older people often worry, worry that cannot be stopped tends to indicate depression. Loneliness when not socially isolated, general rather than specific past regrets, inactivity preceded by a loss of interest, and long pauses before speaking also indicate depression rather than advanced old age" (Kermis, 1986, p. 195). The impression one gets when interacting with a depressed older person is that the individual is "stuck," is unable to decide whether to say something or not or to do something or not.

Depressed people are often confused, but they may or may not be cognitively impaired, and it is difficult to differentiate which is the cart and which is the horse in this regard. Depression goes hand in hand with many illnesses that may be dementing, especially stroke. Persons who are depressed may not try as hard in performing mental tasks, and they may simply be apathetic rather than demented. Depressed people are more likely to complain of memory loss than are those with true dementia. Older depressed people may be more likely to experience weight loss and show **paranoid** symptoms, fears and suspicions that have no basis in fact. They are less likely to express guilt and report feeling depressed than are younger people with depression (Gomez and Gomez, 1993).

The criteria for major depression include poor appetite, sleep disturbances, restlessness, exhaustion, loss of pleasure in activities, feelings of guilt or worthlessness, diminished ability to concentrate, and recurrent thoughts of suicide. Depression is sometimes called the common cold of emotional illness in later life because of its frequency, especially among the isolated aged (Figure 2-5). Epidemiological studies of the elderly have found 2.4 percent to be clinically depressed and another 5.6 percent to be moderately depressed (Stephenson-Cino et al., 1992). Those who are sick for other reasons, of course, may be more likely to also be depressed, and it is common for older persons who are hospitalized for physical problems to show signs of depression. Depression is one of the affective disorders that can be successfully treated, usually with mood-elevating drugs.

Bipolar Disorder.   **Bipolar disorder** is another affective disorder. If a depressed person has ever had a **manic** episode, then the condition can be classified as bipolar. This disorder used to be called manic-depressive illness. It is characterized by mood swings. Alternating with depression are periods where the individual cannot stop talking, sleeps less, is impulsive and irritable, and has confused thoughts. Periods of mania begin suddenly and escalate rapidly; they may last from a few days to several months. Older people with bipolar disorder generally stay disturbed longer than younger ones, and they may seem more confused, paranoid, and agitated. Criteria for diagnosis include increased activity, restlessness, increased talking, flights of ideas, inflated self-esteem, decreased attention span, and excessive involvement in activities that have a high potential for painful consequences. This can include buying sprees, sexual indiscretions, foolish business investments, or reckless driving. Bipolar disorder is treated much like depression, but it has the potential to be more long-lasting.

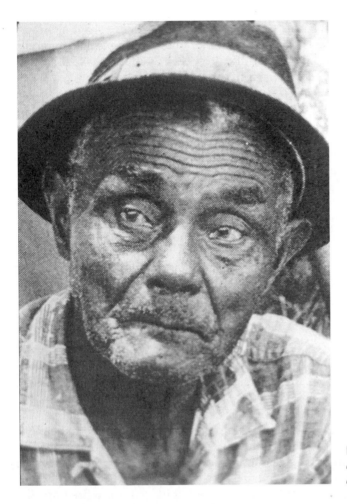

Figure 2-5 *Depression is the most common emotional problem of isolated elders.*

Paraphrenia. **Paraphrenia** refers to delusional disorders of older people, although the term now seems more common in Great Britain. In the United States, those with a well-organized system of paranoid delusions or hallucinations are more likely to be described as being schizophrenic with delusional or paranoid disorders. Unlike true schizophrenia, however, late-onset paraphrenia usually has few negative symptoms. The individual has an intact personality and a normal affective response. Paraphrenia is probably an appropriate term for those in later life who have mild delusions; these are sometimes associated with hearing loss. People with paraphrenia generally have thoughts that are fairly harmless, but they can be dangerous in some instances. Those who fill their houses to overflowing with useless items they feel are of some value, often creating little more than a fire trap, may have late-life paraphrenia.

Paranoid disorder. The basic features of paranoid disorder are irrational thoughts or delusions, including resentment and anger that may lead to violence. The truly paranoid older person often is so eccentric as to have become socially isolated. He or she is often suspicious, and this suspicion is often focused on one or two individuals. People with paranoid disorder are often hostile, angry people who are difficult to work with. They have driven off family and friends and often can be found in circumstances of serious self-neglect.

Schizophrenia.   Schizophrenia is at the extreme along a continuum of mental illnesses, and it affects cognition and reasoning ability in all cases. Schizophrenia is characterized by gross loss of contact with the outer world, deterioration of functioning, and disintegration of personality. It often involves hallucinations and social isolation associated with paranoia. Schizophrenics have markedly peculiar behavior, such as collecting trash, talking to themselves in public, hoarding things, and driving off others. Whereas persons with paraphrenia may actually intend to read the pile of newspapers crowding them out of the living room, persons with schizophrenia may collect actual garbage with no particular thought for an ultimate use. They in fact may not be aware that they are collecting trash. They may also have inappropriate responses, such as laughing or crying that is unrelated to their circumstances. Schizophrenia may be present along with mental retardation. There are few cases of new schizophrenia in later life: "Those individuals who are schizophrenic are predominantly chronic, 'burnt out' cases who manifest the symptoms of 'institutionalism' rather than schizophrenia" (Kermis, 1986, p. 188). Chronic schizophrenia can be dementing, either because of the disease itself or because of the high-powered drugs used to treat it over the course of years.

CASE STUDY

Myrtle Downs continually battled with her sons and daughters. They wanted to help her clean out her home, which she had filled to overflowing with items she brought home from garage sales. She argued that many of the treasures she acquired would appreciate in value over the years. Her children pointed out that any real collectibles would be crushed under the weight of the accumulated junk in Myrtle's house. And, it indeed was a fire trap. She had several years of stacked newspapers that she intended to read. There were little trails through the various rooms in her house between papers and magazines stacked to eye level and beyond. She worked in a hobby store prior to her retirement, and there were boxes and boxes of crafts she intended to make some day. She had literally thousands of shoes and hundreds of dresses piled up throughout the house. In fact, she was not able to sleep in her bed because of the piles of clutter; she slept in a reclining chair at the end of one of the paths in the living room. One bedroom was devoted almost entirely to magazines and books. Her two sons finally persuaded her that the house was a hazard. After filling three dumpsters with trash, the house was in a reasonable semblance of order.

It took Myrtle almost the entire next winter to fill it up again.

WORKING WITH CONFUSED OLDER PEOPLE

There are a number of implications for working with delusional, demented, and depressed older people. Patients who have a cognitive impairment have a problem taking in, processing, and remembering information. Teaching them new things may be exceedingly difficult. However, there are a few things that might help in dealing with confusion in later life (Thorson, 1995):

1. Provide structured routines. Base the sequence of treatment as closely as possible on the patient's normal daily routines. It may be necessary to get information on habits and typical behaviors from family members.
2. Clearly label things. Place identifying labels on the patient's equipment, as well as on his room, closet, bathroom, and personal items.
3. Use familiar items. Ask the family to bring in personal items that are familiar to the individual.
4. Never surprise the patient. Always approach people with a dementing condition from the front, move slowly, and never touch without speaking first.
5. Always orient the patient. Begin and end conversations with orienting information. Always introduce yourself and explain what it is you are going to do.
6. Always use a calm and gentle approach. Even seriously demented people can tell the difference between positive and hostile communication.
7. Be as clear as possible. When communicating with a person with dementia, speak clearly and use short, simple sentences and words. Give only one direction at a time, and allow time for the individual to respond.
8. Maximize internal control and independence. Offer realistic choices whenever possible.
9. Use positive reinforcement. Always praise the patient when he or she completes a task successfully.

Many geriatric patients lose function while in the hospital, so minimizing the length of stay is critical. This goal is difficult to achieve, however, especially among those who are demented or delirious. For the respiratory care practitioner, one implication may be difficulty in the administration of breathing treatments. While younger patients can be left with a mask over the face, this is not the case with the cognitively impaired older adult. UCLA clinician Rebecca Heffler is quoted in a recent article: " 'The second you turn your back, the patient may remove the face mask,' she explains. 'When dementia or delirium is involved, the patient may not understand what the mask is for and will yank it off out of fright. Others will take the mask off and begin talking to it as if it were another person. With these patients, it is necessary to stay right there with them at bedside to help them through the treatment' " (Smith, 1995, p. 36). The point is also made that treatments via metered-dose inhalers require special assistance, as many older people lack the coordination to self-administer the medications.

SUMMARY

Total care of geriatric patients means becoming aware of psychosocial issues that influence their well-being and their treatment. Physical conditions are intimately associated with social and psychological issues. A depressed person, a man who has just lost his wife, a woman who has just experienced the death of a grandchild, an individual who has recently been placed in a nursing home—all of these people have things going on in their lives that will affect their response to treatment.

Some older people may not seem to try as hard to achieve the same goals expected among younger patients. If they are depressed, they may be ambivalent as to whether or not they actually want to get well, or they may not be able to focus on tasks demanded of them. Those going through a life review may find that explaining themselves to others might be more important than taking direction or advice from health care practitioners. Learning new things—especially things that may seem to be pretty high-tech to them—may take extra time and repetition. People with dementia often require constant monitoring.

On the positive side, many older people are repositories of wisdom. They may share interesting experiences and lessons from life. They may be inspiring in the ways that they cope with adversity. People who have lived full, rich lives may be able to teach us things we never expected if we take the time to value the things that the elderly have to share with us.

Review Questions

1. What are some of the social losses you have seen among older people you know?
2. Describe how the exchange theory works between younger and middle-aged adults.
3. We expect personality to remain pretty much of a constant over time. What factors might change it?
4. Have you seen anyone with stress overload (or experienced it yourself)? What happened, and what seemed to help?
5. Describe some of the ways to minimize sick role behavior among older patients.
6. What are some things therapists can do to encourage life reviewing?
7. What behaviors seem to be different among people with Alzheimer's disease as compared to people with multi-infarct dementia?

References

Beard, B. B. (1968). Some characteristics of recent memory of centenarians. *Journal of Gerontology 23*, 23–30.

Bell, B. C., Kara, G., and Batterson, C. (1978). Service utilization and adjustment patterns of elderly tornado victims in an American disaster. *Mass Emergencies, 3*, 71–81.

Brayne, C. (1993). Research and Alzheimer's disease: An epidemiological perspective. *Psychological Medicine, 23*, 287–296.

Butler, R. N. (1963). The life review: An interpretation of reminiscence in the aged. *Psychiatry, 26*, 65–76.

Gomez, G. E., and Gomez, E. A. (1993). Depression in the elderly. *Journal of Psychosocial Nursing, 31* (5), 28–33.

Hagestad, G. O., and Neugarten, B. L. (1985). Age and the life course. In R. H. Binstock and E. Shanas (Eds.), *Handbook of aging and the social sciences,* 2nd ed. New York: Van Nostrand Reinhold, pp. 35–61.

Holmes, T. H., and Rahe, R. H. (1967). The social readjustment rating scale. *Journal of Psychosomatic Research, 11,* 213–218.

Johnson, C. L., and Troll, L. (1992). Family functioning in late late life. *Journal of Gerontology: Social Sciences, 47,* S66–72.

Kermis, M. D. (1986). *Mental health in late life.* Boston: Jones & Bartlett.

Poon, L. W., Messner, S., Martin, P., Noble, C. A., Clayton, G., and Johnson, M. A. (1992). The influences of cognitive resources on adaptation and old age. *International Journal of Aging and Human Development, 24,* 31–46.

Seligman, M. E. P. (1975). *Helplessness.* San Francisco: Freeman.

Smith, R. (1995). Elder-care's shining example. *RT—The Journal for Respiratory Care Practitioners, 8* (1), 33–36.

Steinbach, U. (1992). Social networks, institutionalization, and mortality among elderly people in the United States. *Journal of Gerontology: Social Sciences, 47,* S183–190.

Stephenson-Cino, P., Steiner, M., Krames, L., Ryan, E. B., et al. (1992). Depression in elderly persons and its correlates in family practice: A Canadian study. *Psychological Reports, 70,* 359–368.

Stinnet, N., and DeFrain, J. D. (1985). *Secrets of strong families.* Boston: Little, Brown.

Thorson, J. A. (1988). Relocation of the elderly: Some implications from the research. *Gerontology Review, 1* (1), 28–36.

Thorson, J. A. (1995). *Aging in a changing society.* Belmont, CA: Wadsworth.

Thorson, J. A., and Powell, F. C. (1990). Meanings of death and intrinsic religiosity. *Journal of Clinical Psychology, 46,* 379–391.

Thorson, J. A., and Thorson, J. R. (1981). Keeping the older person alive. In L. H. Andrus, M. O'Hara-Devereaux, and C. Scott (Eds.), *A practical guide to clinical geriatrics.* New York: Grune & Stratton, pp. 331–335.

Thorson, J. A., and Thorson, J. R. (1986). How accurate are stress scales? *Journal of Gerontological Nursing, 12* (1), 21–24.

U. S. Bureau of the Census (1995). *Statistical Abstract of the United States.* Washington, DC: U. S. Government Printing Office.

Vaillant, G. E. (1977). *Adaptation to life.* Boston: Little, Brown.

CHAPTER THREE

ANATOMIC AND PHYSIOLOGIC CHANGES IN LATER LIFE

——————————— KEY TERMS ———————————

activities of daily living
autoimmune
biological clock
closing capacity
closing volume
cross-linking theory
endocrine theory

error catastrophe theory
error theories
evolutionary model
free radical theory
genetic program
hypercapnia
hypoxemia

hypoxia
immunological theory
lamina propria
programmed theories
rate of living theory
somatic mutation theory
wear and tear theory

——————————— LEARNING OBJECTIVES ———————————

After completing this chapter, the reader should be able to:

1. Describe basic physical models of the aging process.
2. Differentiate error theories of aging from programmed theories of aging.
3. Describe how older persons tend to use functional capacity as an index of personal health.
4. List some of the age-related changes in the trachea, bronchi, and alveoli.
5. Describe how pulmonary function testing might differ among aged individuals.

INTRODUCTION

At the most basic physical level, aging can be characterized as loss of cells and slowing of cellular function. These changes are manifested in slowing processes in the aging body, a decline in the functioning of the immune system, increasing morbidity, and the ultimate failure of one or more physical systems, resulting in death. These concepts are universal. However, very few people die of old age itself. The majority of the population dies in late life, and most people die of a disease associated with old age. Chronic killers such as heart disease, cancer, and cerebrovascular diseases are much more common in later life. Pneumonia and chronic obstructive pulmonary diseases are major killers of the elderly. Other than the unnatural causes of death—accidents, suicide, and homicide—the processes of aging can be seen as underlying most causes of mortality.

It is explained in Chapter 1 how the survival curve becomes increasingly steep later in life. Most of the human population dies between ages 65 and 85. Only 3 out of 10,000 live to age 100, and it takes over a million 100-year-olds to produce even one who lives to 110 (Thorson, 1995). Almost all older people die from a disease or definable physical process, most of which can be attributed to declining responses associated with biological aging.

BIOLOGICAL CAUSES OF AGING

It might be said that people are programmed to develop, age, and die. Children's baby teeth are replaced by 5 or 6 years of age, and they acquire a new set of molars at the same time. Nearly every child enters puberty at about age 12, plus or minus a year or two. Most people begin to observe a few gray hairs in their fourth decade of life; at the same time, their eyes typically change shape and they may have difficulty focusing at close distances. Women cease to menstruate in the fifth decade of life. Seeing these changes happen over time like **biological clockwork,** it is fair to conclude that the length of life is biologically programmed as well.

INEVITABILITY OF AGING AS A PHYSICAL PROCESS

Cross-linkages of cells and the replacement of muscle with connective tissue characterize the physical aging of all animals. This is the reason that meat from an older animal is tough and meat from a young one is tender. Added to this toughening is a drying process: the older body has from 7 to 12 percent less water than a young body. In humans, there is a movement of body fat from just under the skin to the middle of the body, which is one of the reasons for wrinkling. There is a migration of subcutaneous fat that once kept young people's skin smooth and insulated their bodies against heat and cold. Bone begins to lose its integrity and becomes more porous. There is a decline in sensory perception. Overall speed, strength, and reserve capacity decline, as does the efficiency of all organ systems and the immune system.

Aging is as inexorable as gravity. Humans are socialized to recognize the signs of physical aging. Being able to describe a process, however, is different from explaining why it occurs. Throughout recorded history there are examples of human struggles with mortality, with the inevitable decline that comes with the processes of physical aging. It is only recently, however, that scientists have begun to understand some of the underlying reasons for biological changes associated with the aging process. Unfortunately, there is no universally accepted model of physical aging; instead, there are a number of theories of aging, all of which may be correct to one degree or another.

CALORIC RESTRICTION MODEL

It has been known since the 1930s that the lives of laboratory rats and mice can be extended by feeding them a nutritionally complete diet but restricting their overall caloric intake (McCay, Crowell, and Maynard, 1935). It is generally known that an effective way of producing a population of really old laboratory rats is to feed them every other day. Whether or not this effect occurs in higher animals has not been determined. It is clear, though, that food restriction in rodents does in fact retard the basic biological processes of aging and extends their lives about 40 to 50 percent. Currently there is no single adequate explanation for this finding.

There is an alteration of the glycation reactions that take place with the metabolism of food (Masoro, Katz, and McMahan, 1989). Still, an explanation of this response does not provide an adequate description of why aging itself takes place. Underlying causes of aging are still theoretical. There may be many different underlying causes of physical aging. There are two principal groups of biological theories of aging: **error theories** and **programmed theories.**

ERROR THEORIES OF AGING

The error theories are mainly descriptive—they rely on observation. The **wear and tear theory,** for example, simply recognizes that cells and tissues, when exposed to a variety of environmental stresses, wear out eventually just like a set of tires on a car. Unlike a set of tires, however, the body actively repairs and replaces itself, bit by bit. It is this process of regeneration and replacement that gradually fails, thus causing signs of physical aging. This is an adequate description of biological aging, but it is not an adequate explanation of why it takes place. Related to the wear and tear theory is the **rate of living theory;** it says that the greater the organism's rate of oxygen metabolism, the shorter the life span. This theory might explain why the Galapagos tortoise has a life of 150 years and a shrew has a span of under a year, but the theory breaks down when other animals are observed. Why, for example, do swans and parrots often live for over 50 years, yet pandas seldom live as long as 15? It is apparent that the idea that living fast and burning out has some validity, but it is not an adequate explanation of the process of aging itself.

More complex error theories accept this rate of living hypothesis, but add that collagen accumulates in older bodies. This **cross-linking theory** of aging holds that glucose molecules attach themselves to proteins, causing them to cross-link and damage cells and eventually slow down bodily processes.

There are two additional error theories. The **error catastrophe theory** says that faulty proteins accumulate to such a level as to cause damage to cells. The **somatic mutation the-**

ory holds that the accumulation of genetic mutations over time causes cell malfunctions that lead to the aging of the organism. It is both an error theory and an additional type of explanation of biological aging, a programmed theory.

PROGRAMMED THEORIES OF AGING

Programmed theories of aging hold that the life span of a species is programmed genetically, which has been demonstrated in the laboratory. Prior to the early 1960s it had been thought that plant and animal cells could divide indefinitely. A project that began early in the twentieth century had kept chicken fibroblasts alive in the laboratory for many years longer than the life span of chickens as a species (Carrel and Burrows, 1911). This project was taken as proof that the essential biological process of aging was not at the cellular level but had to be higher, at the tissue or the organ level, for instance. However, repeated attempts to replicate this experiment have failed, and it is presumed that in some way new live cells had been introduced into the medium when the experimental cultures were fed.

In the late 1950s, a series of experiments on causes of cancer led to a finding on the programmed basis of genetic aging that contradicted the earlier research. It was necessary to grow human fetal tissue in a laboratory setting in order to conduct this research. These normal cell populations grew and doubled for many months. Then they slowed down, stopped, and died. The only cells that continued doubling without limit were cancerous.

After repeated studies, it became evident that a kind of biological time clock programmed the aging process and dictated the life span of cells in laboratory culture and in living creatures as well. Embryonic cells grew and doubled about fifty times. Cells taken from young adults would double only about thirty times before they ceased and died, and cells from older people had about twenty doublings left. Cells that had been frozen and then thawed out after many years retained a genetic memory of how many times they had doubled. They picked up where they had left off (Hayflick, 1974).

This research has been replicated many times in many different laboratories throughout the world. Different species have a different number of cell doublings programmed into their basic genetic structure. This finding supports the theory that cells have a **genetic program** to replace themselves a set number of times and then cease replication. Leonard Hayflick, the scientist who first discovered this effect, says that in essence we are programmed to die. Few old people, however, ever reach the limit of their number of cell doublings. Almost all die of something else first. This theory explains why humans mature at essentially the same rate. There is genetic information that dictates when basic physical changes occur, when the organism slows down, and ultimately when the cells no longer replace themselves.

The **endocrine theory** of aging is an extension of this theory of programmed senescence. It says that the biological time clock in each cell is activated by hormones to control the pace of the aging process. Hormones are also influential in the functioning of the immune system. The endocrine theory of aging, then, is something of a bridge between the programmed theory and the immunological theory.

The **immunological theory** of aging says that aging of the immune system influences the aging process of the individual (Makinodan, 1977). Most deaths occur because of immune system failure. The thymus, which plays an important role in early life, begins to decrease in size and functioning early in adulthood. There is a reduction in function of T cells, the cells secreted by the thymus gland. There is a loss of cells in the thymic cortex and a corresponding decrease in the excretion of thymic hormone. The result is a programmed decline in immune system functioning.

A related immunological theory says that with aging the body develops more **autoimmune** antibodies that destroy normal cells. The frequency of autoimmune reactions such as arthritis and diabetes increases with aging. A slowing of the functional ability of the immune system to produce antibodies increases the vulnerability of the body to disease. Disease speeds decrements in cellular, tissue, organ, and organ system functioning. Thus, there is an increased susceptibility to both infection and the formation of benign and malignant neoplasms.

The **free radical theory** of aging holds that much of the damage done during the process of aging is chemical and is caused by free radicals in the body. Hydroxyl ions, or molecules containing an unpaired electron, which makes them highly reactive, are produced by oxygen metabolism. Just as in the process of burning, oxygen metabolism produces carbon dioxide, water, and hydroxyl ions. These hydroxyl ions often initiate chain reactions in their efforts to combine with other molecules, and these reactions often produce other free radicals. Such reactions are thought to be the underlying reason for damage to cell membranes and acceleration of the aging process. Free radicals can oxidize virtually all cellular components including nucleic acids and proteins.

Free radicals are usually destroyed by protective enzymes. Studies have shown the effect of antioxidant enzymes, superoxide dismutase and catalase, and antioxidants such as vitamins C and E, selinium, and beta-carotene in protecting against damage from free radicals. Harman (1968) demonstrated that laboratory mice fed antioxidants such as BHT (a food preservative) lived much longer than control populations. It is thought that there is not a failure of protective mechanisms so much as that more and more free radicals slip through the protective processes as the organism ages, ultimately overwhelming it. Free radical damage is related to conditions such as cerebrovascular disease and the formation of malignant neoplasms.

SOMATIC MUTATIONS

The somatic mutation theory of aging combines several of the theories that have been discussed. The genetic basis of aging can be affected by hormonal influences as well as the process of slowing cell replication. The somatic mutation theory is based on the concept that changes in deoxyribonucleic acid (DNA) occur through radiation or miscoding, and that these damaged cells replicate, causing mutations. This process may trigger autoimmune reactions. Mutated cellular function diminishes organ efficiency, and age-associated alterations are seen in the organism.

An **evolutionary model** proposes that genetically controlled repair and maintenance at the cellular level works well up to and through the age of reproductivity. The organism has thus lived long enough to accomplish its evolutionary task and essentially has no purpose thereafter. Although organisms are not really programmed to die, they are not programmed to live much beyond the age required to ensure reproductive success. The evolutionary model is not a theory of the biology of aging—it is actually an expression of an outcome of the programmed and endocrine theories.

It is likely that there are additional explanations of the processes of physical aging at the most basic level. It is also probable that the ones discussed are all correct to one degree or another. It is evident that there is no single cause of biological aging and that several explanations work in concert to describe the changes that take place in organisms as they age.

PHYSICAL CHANGES, MORBIDITY, AND MORTALITY

Individuals seem to age at different rates. Everyone knows people who seem to be old at 60 and those who are still going strong at 85. Within individuals, organ and organ systems show different rates of decline. Within certain parameters, however, everyone seems to be on a schedule of development and decline that is fairly constant.

DECLINE IN ORGAN SYSTEMS

In general, it can be said that the heart grows somewhat larger with age. During exercise, maximal oxygen consumption among men declines by about 10 percent with each decade of life during adulthood and by about 7.5 percent among women. These rates vary slightly from one individual to another. Declining function, however, is the rule rather than the exception.

Maximum breathing capacity declines in most people by about 40 percent between the ages of 20 and 70 years. The brain loses some neurons and others become damaged over time. Overall brain weight declines. However, there is an increase in the number of connections between synapses and a regrowing of extensions, dendrites, and axons that carry messages within the brain. The kidneys become less efficient and the capacity of the bladder declines. Without exercise, overall muscle mass declines by about 22 percent between the ages of 30 and 70. Hearing, especially of high pitches, decreases from 10 years of age onward, and it declines more quickly in men than in women.

Shock (1976) prepared a listing of the approximate percentages of function remaining in the average 75-year-old, given the value found for the average 30-year-old as 100 percent (Table 3-1).

FUNCTIONAL ABILITY

Functional ability is the ability to accomplish the **activities of daily living (ADLs).** Most older people do not feel that their lives are impaired, and there is a tendency for most to rate themselves as more fit than others their same age (Figure 3-1). Rather, what is typically said is something like this: "I don't feel old except when I can't do something." In fact, functional ability is taken by most gerontologists as a good index of health among the aged. It is important to accurately assess relative levels of disability with surveys of ADLs. Table 3-2 is a listing of responses from a random sample of 700 home-dwelling older people (average age = 72 years) taken in a recent survey.

It would seem from the data in Table 3-2 that the older people represented are remarkably free from disability. However, it must be remembered that this was a community-

TABLE 3-1 **Physical Capacity Remaining at Age 75**

Physical Measure	% Capacity Remaining at 75
Brain weight	56
Blood flow to brain	80
Speed of return to equilibrium of blood acidity	17
Cardiac output at rest	70
Kidney filtration rate	69
Kidney plasma flow	50
Number of nerve trunk fibers	63
Nerve conduction velocity	90
Number of taste buds	36
Maximum oxygen uptake (during exercise)	40
Maximum breathing capacity (voluntary)	43
Vital capacity	56
Hand grip	55
Maximum work rate	70
Basal metabolic rate	84

Source: *Nathan Shock (1976). The physiology of aging. In* Human Physiology and the Environment. *San Francisco: W. H. Freeman. p. 244.*

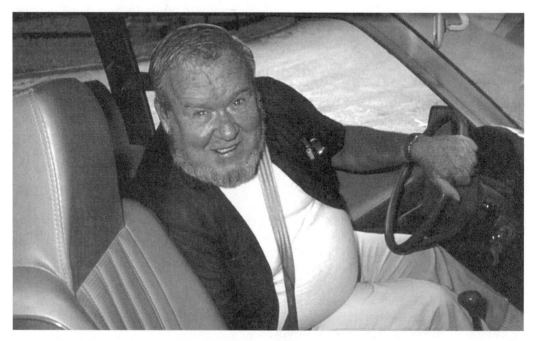

Figure 3-1 *Most older people feel that their lives are not impaired as long as they can do what they want.*

TABLE 3-2   **Survey of ADL Impairments Among a Sample of 700 Older Adults**

Item	Needs Assistance (%)	Cannot Do At All (%)
Can you take a bath or shower?	2.1	0.7
Can you dress and undress yourself?	0.7	0.3
Can you eat?	0.1	0.0
Can you get in and out of bed?	0.4	0.1
Can you walk?	6.4	0.9
Do you ever have trouble getting to the bathroom?	3.4	0.1
Can you prepare your own meals?	2.1	0.7
Can you go shopping?	6.4	2.1
Can you handle your money?	0.5	0.3
Can you do your own housework?	8.7	2.4
Can you get to places out of walking distance of your home?	8.4	1.7

Source: *F. C. Powell and J. A. Thorson (1994)*. Social Conditions of Nebraska's Elderly. *Omaha: Department of Gerontology, University of Nebraska at Omaha.*

dwelling sample. Institutionalized persons were not surveyed. Taken in that context, it appears that about 6 to 8 percent of the aged who live at home can do so only with some assistance. They may need help doing housework or shopping, for example, in order to maintain their independence. It might also be concluded from these data that those who have trouble with certain critical abilities, especially eating and getting to the bathroom, probably have lost their ability to live on their own and have had to be institutionalized.

About 5 percent of the population age 65 and older are in nursing homes at any one time. Obviously, they are the ones who are sickest and most disabled. This institutionalized population is dealt with in greater detail in Chapter 7. Among those community-dwelling elderly still able to live in their own residence, however, the rates of serious disability are actually quite low. In general, rates of disability go up with age, and rates of disability also go up as income goes down. It is reasonable to conclude, then, that the oldest and poorest among the aging population have the highest rates of functional disability.

CASE STUDY

Kathryn, age 81, suffered a heart attack. Nine years earlier she had a stroke that left her minimally disabled. She lived in a senior citizens' condo and depended on her son to do her shopping and drive her to church and to the doctor. Surveyed as to her perception of her health, she checkmarked "excellent." By age 84 she had advanced renal failure, congestive heart failure, and cataracts. Her final hospitalization was for pneumonia, which was cured. Three weeks before her death she learned that a great-niece would be getting married in Mexico the following December and she began making plans to go to the wedding. Kathryn died at age 85; she would have said that she was healthy as long as she could do the things she wanted to do. In terms of ADLs, she felt that as long as she could cook for herself and get to the bathroom by herself, she could live independently. When it became apparent that these abilities could not be restored, she realized that she had come to the end of her life.

MORBIDITY

Morbidity is the incidence of disease, and when speaking of the aging population, an important distinction should be made relative to rates of disease. Acute conditions, often infectious illnesses, have a fairly rapid course. The body either recovers or succumbs to most acute illnesses in short order. Chronic conditions that occur over a longer period of time, such as arthritis or diabetes, are more characteristic of the elderly. Morbidity among the entire population has changed with the introduction in the 1930s of immunization to prevent specific communicable diseases such as diphtheria, whooping cough, and typhoid fever, and later on with inoculations against polio and measles, as well as the development of effective treatments for major acute illnesses such as tuberculosis and rheumatic fever. In fact, some acute diseases have been wiped out. There were only four reported cases of diphtheria in the United States in 1992; at the beginning of the century, diphtheria was among the ten leading causes of death. Smallpox is not even listed among reportable diseases any longer. Major killers of children have been eliminated; the death rate in the United States in the first year of life in the year 1900 was about 160 per 1,000 live births; it has now declined to 7.5 per 1,000. Improved sanitation, control of infection, and prevention of communicable disease have changed the profile of illness and death for the population of much of the world during the twentieth century. A great many deaths used to occur among children and young people from acute conditions; the majority of deaths now take place late in life from chronic conditions.

Despite compromised immune systems, older people have had more time to develop immunity to many infectious illnesses. The rate of the four most common categories of acute conditions declines with age (Table 3-3). Older people are simply less prone to acquire infectious illness. In what may seem to be a paradox, however, those in frail health who do get a communicable disease are much more likely to die from it. Children are much more likely than older people to have an infective or parasitic acute condition, they are much more likely to have a cold or the flu, and they are much more likely to have an acute condition related to the digestive system (typically, diarrhea). Although the immune system often fails in very late life, most people 65 and older have built up an immunity to everyday pathogens in the environment. Another less optimistic explanation for these lower rates of morbidity from acute causes among the elderly is that those more prone to acquire acute illnesses may have died from one of them prior to reaching old age.

Chronic conditions increase dramatically with age (Table 3-4). Interestingly, prevalence rates at age 75 for chronic bronchitis and asthma are among the few chronic conditions that are not significantly higher than rates for younger adults. Again, it is possible that there has

TABLE 3-3   **Acute Conditions by Age**

Age Group	Rate per 100 Population			
	Infective and Parasitic	**Common Cold**	**Influenza**	**Digestive System**
Total Population	22.4	25.7	42.7	7.0
Under 5 years of age	59.0	66.1	56.7	12.9
5 to 17 years of age	45.2	35.4	59.1	9.2
18 to 24 years of age	20.9	29.6	41.8	5.2
25 to 44 years of age	16.2	21.1	45.7	5.8
45 to 64 years of age	7.1	13.0	31.5	4.7
65 years and older	5.8	14.2	19.1	8.0

Source: *U.S. Bureau of the Census (1994).* Statistical Abstract of the United States, *114th ed.,* Washington, DC.

TABLE 3-4   **Prevalence of Chronic Conditions by Age and Sex, Rate per 100**

Chronic Condition	Under 45	45–64	65–74	75+
Males				
Arthritis	2.6	19.9	36.5	42.7
Cataracts	0.2	1.8	11.2	19.3
Hearing impairments	4.3	21.6	32.2	45.3
Orthopedic impairments	10.2	18.2	15.5	18.6
Diabetes	0.6	5.3	11.9	9.7
Heart conditions	2.6	15.1	33.5	40.8
Hypertension	3.7	23.1	34.1	31.4
Chronic bronchitis	4.1	4.4	7.7	4.0
Asthma	5.1	3.2	2.9	3.6
Females				
Arthritis	4.2	31.6	50.8	61.1
Cataracts	0.2	3.2	13.7	24.5
Hearing impairments	3.4	9.7	20.4	39.3
Orthopedic impairments	10.0	16.7	16+	24.3
Diabetes	0.9	5.9	10.9	11.0
Heart conditions	3.3	12.0	22.1	40.1
Hypertension	3.0	22.2	37.7	37.4
Chronic bronchitis	5.8	7.2	8.0	6.6
Asthma	5.4	5.6	5.6	3.3

Source: *U.S. Bureau of the Census (1994).* Statistical Abstract of the United States, *114th ed.,* Washington, DC.

been a "weeding out" effect—that many people who had these particular chronic conditions have not lived to be counted among those age 75 and older.

Most other chronic illnesses, however, are more prevalent late in life, which means that many elderly people are among the "walking wounded," and that the typical older person has several chronic health problems. One implication is that the so-called medical model of treatment and cure of acute illness is less applicable for the principal health problems found among members of the older population. Their health problems are not prone to cure but instead to management. Diseases such as diabetes, hypertension, and arthritis will likely be with individuals for the rest of their lives. They may not be cured, but they can be managed with greater or lesser success. There are many older people who have a number of serious, potentially fatal, chronic conditions who rate their health as good or excellent because these conditions are effectively under control. This careful management of chronic conditions is the goal of geriatric medicine.

MORTALITY

Causes of mortality, like morbidity, change over the course of the life span. It is the case, however, that many of the chronic conditions from which older people suffer are not necessarily the cause of their death. No one really dies from arthritis or cataracts. But there is some evidence that many people in frail health who may suffer from major chronic illness ultimately succumb to an acute infection.

It is sobering to realize in these days of faith in science and medicine that the digest of causes of death found in the *Monthly Vital Statistics Report* issued by the U.S. Centers for Disease Control invariably lists "symptoms, signs, and ill-defined conditions" and "all other diseases" combined as accounting for about 10 percent of the total. That is, the causes of about one in ten deaths are indeterminate. Even less heartening is the fact that from 20 to 30 percent of autopsies invariably find a cause of death different from what the individual was being treated for (Thorson, 1995).

Still, the leading causes of death throughout the population are chronic conditions (Table 3-5). People of different ages, however, die of different things. Children under 5 years of age account for only three-tenths of 1 percent of the total deaths in any one year— slightly over 7,000 out of about 2.4 million. Their leading causes of death are accidents, birth defects (congenital anomalies), cancer, homicide, heart disease, and pneumonia. By young adulthood, the leading causes of death have shifted to accidents, homicide, and suicide.

Of the approximately 1.6 million people 65 and over who die each year, the leading causes are heart disease (38 percent), cancer (23 percent), cerebrovascular disease or stroke (8 percent), chronic obstructive pulmonary disease (5 percent), and pneumonia and influenza (4.5 percent). Again, it can be seen that the group representing by far the greatest number and percentage of deaths, the aged, dies mostly from chronic conditions. Chapter 8 goes into greater detail on the changes in death that have taken place during the twentieth century.

There are more detailed mortality data of particular interest to respiratory care practitioners. Death rates for chronic obstructive pulmonary disease as well as for pneumonia and influenza increase greatly late in life (Table 3-6).

TABLE 3-5 Causes of Death in Percentages

Cause	Percent of Total Deaths
Heart diseases	32.6
Malignant neoplasms	23.4
Cerebrovascular diseases	6.8
Chronic obstructive pulmonary diseases	4.5
Accidents	3.9
Pneumonia and influenza	3.5
Diabetes mellitus	2.6
HIV (human immunodeficiency virus) infection	1.5
Suicide	1.3
Nephritis	1.1
Birth defects	1.0
Chronic liver disease and cirrhosis	1.0
Homicide	0.9
Septicemia	0.9
Atherosclerosis	0.7
All other causes	14.3

Source: *U.S. Centers for Disease Control (1997)*. Monthly Vital Statistics Report, *April 24, 45 (10).*

TABLE 3-6 Deaths from Chronic Obstructive Pulmonary Diseases and from Pneumonia and Influenza, by Age and Sex, Rates per 100,000 Population

	Death Rates					
	All Ages	45–54 Years	55–64 Years	65–74 Years	75–84 Years	85 Years and Older
Chronic Obstructive Pulmonary Diseases						
Male	43.4	8.4	61.9	205.2	524.7	864.7
Female	35.1	8.5	42.6	134.5	264.9	336.6
Pneumonia and Influenza						
Male	29.6	7.6	23.0	75.4	329.1	1,315.0
Female	33.6	5.1	14.3	40.0	186.7	1,002.1

Source: *U.S. Centers for Disease Control (1994)*. Monthly Vital Statistics Report, *October 11. Vol. 42, No. 13.*

About 8 percent of all deaths are accounted for by chronic obstructive pulmonary disease, pneumonia, and influenza, totaling 188,284 individuals in 1995 (Centers for Disease Control, 1996). Rates of death from these conditions increase dramatically with age, reaching their highest rate among the population age 85 and older. The other principal pulmonary disease that is a major killer is lung cancer, accounting for 156,073 deaths that year, or 6.7 percent of the total.

PULMONARY CHANGES ASSOCIATED WITH AGING

Aging is a normal, progressive, and physiologically irreversible process (Des Jardins, 1993). The rate of aging varies among individuals, but it nevertheless proceeds in spite of genetics, the environment, a healthy diet, or daily exercise. A gradual decline in muscle strength, skin elasticity, blood circulation, and sensory acuity are noted with increasing age. It could be said that about a quarter of life is spent growing up and the remaining three quarters is spent growing old. A common sign of aging is failure of the individual to maintain as high a level of physical activity as was once possible. Decremental changes in the muscular and circulatory systems contribute to the overall decline, but a major cause of reduced functional ability is the decreased capability of the respiratory system to acquire and deliver oxygen to the arterial blood (Spence, 1989). This impairment in oxygen delivery is the end result of many age-related changes in the pulmonary system.

AGE-RELATED CHANGES

There are a number of age-related changes in the physiology of the pulmonary system, including the trachea and bronchi, the alveoli, and the lungs themselves.

Trachea and Bronchi.   The trachea and bronchi change over the course of the life cycle. Progressive calcification of cartilage in the walls of the trachea and bronchi causes increased rigidity with aging. The smooth muscle fibers found in the **lamina propria,** the submucosal layer of the tracheobronchial tree, tend to be replaced with fibrous connective tissue. The distensibility of the bronchioles is reduced. With increasing age, the epithelial cells of the mucous membrane that line the tracheobronchial tree show degenerative changes. Ciliary activity slows down. There is a decrease in the phagocytic activity of the macrophages in the mucous membrane. Combined, these changes all lead to a reduction in mucocillary clearance.

Anatomic dead space—the internal volume of the conducting airways, from the nose and mouth down to, but not including, the gas exchange units—also increases slightly with age. This change probably reflects loss of elasticity and increased lung volume rather than a direct effect on the large airways (Slonim and Hamilton, 1987).

Alveoli.   Alveoli change functionally. At birth, infants have about 24 million rudimentary alveoli (Lough, Doershuk, and Stern, 1985). Alveoli continue to form throughout childhood. Although most investigators seem to agree that the majority of alveoli develop after birth, exactly when alveolar multiplication ends has yet to be determined. Estimates are that the maximum number of alveoli have been formed between 5 and 8 years of age. The alveolar number in adults has been estimated at approximately 300 million, depending on body size (Lough, Doershuk, and Stern, 1985).

The number of alveoli remains essentially constant throughout old age, but there is a gradual deterioration of the alveolar septa. Loss of alveolar walls increases the size of the alveoli and reduces the surface area available for gas diffusion. Cross-linkages develop between collagen fibers in the alveolar walls, which limits the expansion of the alveoli during inspiration. The structural change that occurs during the course of aging is an increased diameter of the alveolar ducts, and as a result the alveoli arising from them are wider and shallower (Murray, 1986).

Lungs. The lungs are subject to many age-related changes. The growth of the lungs is essentially complete by age 20 (Des Jardins, 1993). As adults age there is a progressive loss of alveolar elastic recoil. This loss of elasticity seems to result more from alterations in composition of the elastic and collagen fibers than from an actual reduction of elastic fibers. Conversely, it has been reported that the amount of elastic fibers in the lung increases with age (Spence, 1989). One possibility is that pseudoelastin is present in aging human lungs and gives a deceptively elevated elastin content, as measured by chemical analysis (Ranga, Kleinerman, and Sorensen, 1979). Nevertheless, aging lungs have lost elastic recoil and offer less resistance to expansion. There is also an increase in the stiffness of the thoracic cage due to calcification of the costal cartilage.

Age-related bone loss, leading to decreased spaces between the spinal vertebrae and a greater degree of spinal curvature, is an additional factor leading to decreased chest wall compliance (Levitzky, Cairo, and Hall, 1990). Ultimately, these changes in elastic recoil and stiffness of the thoracic cage shift the end-expiratory position upward, thus increasing the functional residual capacity (Martin and Youtsey, 1988). The work necessary to overcome these static mechanical alterations is estimated to be 20 percent higher for a 60-year-old than for an individual who is 20 years of age (Des Jardins, 1993).

The increased work to move air in and out of the lungs causes some older people to rely more on the diaphragm for inspiration. The contraction and expansion of the diaphragm, however, can be affected by intra-abdominal pressure. Lying on the back increases intra-abdominal pressure. Elderly people may find it easier to breathe if their upper body is elevated as opposed to being supine.

Despite alterations in their structure and function, the lungs appear to be relatively durable. Unless affected by disease, they are capable of maintaining adequate gas exchange for the maximum life span (Murray, 1986).

Pulmonary function gradually declines in adults after the age of 25. The age-related changes in lung volumes and capacities are in a downward direction (Figure 3-2).

The effect of senescence on pulmonary function measurements has been well documented. When trying to diagnose functional impairment from pulmonary disease by performing pulmonary function testing in the elderly, it is important that age-appropriate norms be used as the standard. Aging alone will cause the following pulmonary function changes:

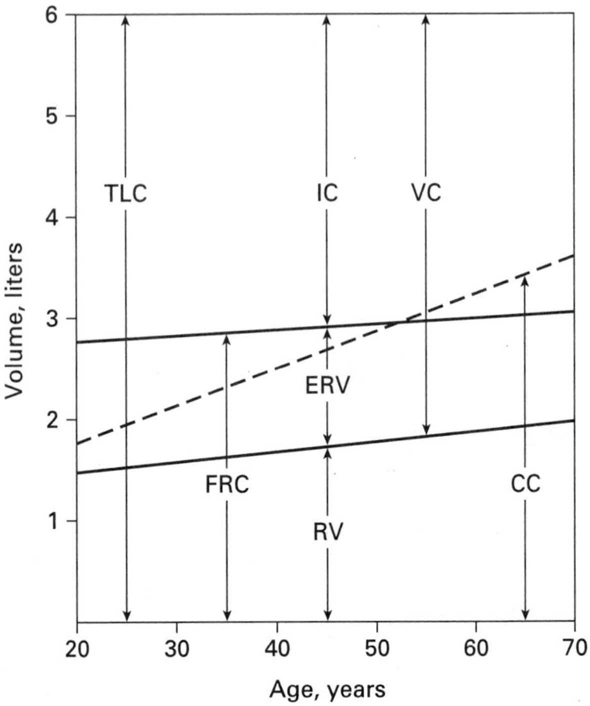

Figure 3-2 *Alterations in the standard lung volumes and capacities occurring with age. TLC = total lung capacity, FRC = functional residual capacity, ERV = expiratory reserve volume, RV = residual volume, IC = inspiratory capacity, VC = vital capacity, CC = closing capacity.* (Source: *M. G. Levitzky,* Pulmonary physiology, *3rd ed. New York: McGraw-Hill. Reprinted by permission.)*

- Reduced vital capacity, both slow and forced
- Reduced peak expiratory flows
- Reduced inspiratory capacity
- Reduced forced expiratory flows ($FEF_{25-75\%}$)
- Reduced forced expiratory volume in 1 second (FEV_1)
- Decreased diffusing capacity
- Increased residual volume
- Increased functional residual capacity

To comprehend these pulmonary function variations, refer back to the age-related changes in the lungs and alveoli, including loss of elastic recoil, loss of alveolar surface area, and collagen fiber alterations.

Overall lung compliance decreases in the older adult. The loss of elasticity actually increases lung compliance. The cross-linkages of the collagen fibers in the alveolar walls, however, in addition to the calcification of costal cartilage, causing decreased chest wall compliance, result in a net reduction of lung compliance.

The effect of changes in lung and chest wall mechanics cause forced vital capacity (FVC) and FEV_1 to diminish as early as age 25. The mean rate of decline is approximately 32 milliliters per year for men and 25 milliliters per year for women (Lamy, 1980). The residual volume increases almost 50 percent by age 70 (Murray, 1986).

The total lung capacity remains relatively stable in elderly patients, especially when related to height. Tidal volume and respiratory rate also remain reasonably constant. When exertion mandates an increased minute ventilation, it is usually the rate of breathing that increases, not the tidal volume.

PULMONARY FUNCTION TESTING

Standard pulmonary function testing in the elderly requires significant coordination and cooperation on the part of the patient and the therapist. Explaining the procedure to the patient may take longer and require more demonstration. Frequent maneuvers, such as repeated breath holding and timed effort-dependent exhalations with maximal breathing effort are required. All of these may be difficult to perform and may provide unreliable results in older or debilitated patients (Chalker and Celli, 1993). After obtaining the best data possible, a note to the pulmonologist concerning the patient's level of comprehension and performance may help assist in the interpretation of the results.

Chalker and Celli (1993) describe forced oscillation, which is an independent means of measuring pulmonary function. In an effort-independent maneuver, short bursts of sound from a simple loudspeaker measure the movement of air in and out of the lungs while the patient does tidal breathing through a mouthpiece. The use of forced oscillation to measure respiratory system impedance may have a future role in assessing elderly patients who have difficulty performing standard pulmonary function testing maneuvers.

PULMONARY GAS EXCHANGE

Gas exchange is altered to a certain degree among the elderly. Ventilation/perfusion inequalities, normally due to anatomic shunts and regional differences in ventilation and perfusion, are even more pronounced in older adults.

Physiological shunt increases from less than 5 percent at age 20 to about 15 percent at age 70 (Levitzky, 1991). As was noted earlier, the age-related loss of alveolar surface area also reduces diffusing capacity. Pulmonary diffusing capacity (D_LCO) decreases progressively and linearly over time, falling approximately 20 percent over the course of adult life (Levitzky, 1991). Another factor in reduced D_LCO is decreased pulmonary capillary blood flow, which is a consequence of both the age-related alveolar changes and the reduced cardiac index in the aged.

Loss of elastic recoil creates other problems for the elderly. Static compliance, which is the inverse of elastic recoil, increases with age. Changes in **closing volume** and **closing capacity** affect gas exchange. Closing volume is the volume of gas in the lungs in excess of residual volume that remains when small airways in the dependent lower portions of the lungs close during maximal exhalation. Closing capacity is simply closing volume plus residual volume. The closing capacity increases from about 30 percent of the total lung capacity (TLC) at age 20 to about 58 percent of TLC at age 70 (Figure 3-2; Levitzky, Cairo, and

Hall, 1990). The loss of elastic recoil results in decreased support of small airways, which leads to early airway closure in the elderly. Closure reduces ventilation to the lower lung regions and shifts the distribution of ventilation to the upper lung regions. Perfusion, or blood flow, increases only slightly in the upper lung regions of aged lungs, with the majority of blood flow still perfusing the lower lung regions. These physiological alterations—ventilation to upper lung segments, perfusion to lower lung segments—result in a ventilation/perfusion mismatch larger than normal.

OXYGENATION

Arterial partial pressure of oxygen (PaO_2) declines with aging. The resting PaO_2 can be estimated by the following equations (Tierney, McPhee, and Papadakis, 1995):

$$PaO_2 = 104 - (Age \times 0.42) \text{ supine}$$
$$PaO_2 = 104 - (Age \times 0.27) \text{ sitting}$$

Alveolar partial pressure of oxygen (PAO_2) remains relatively stable throughout the aging process, leading to an elevated alveolar-arterial (A-a) O_2 gradient (Levitzky, 1991). This elevated (A-a) O_2 gradient in the elderly is probably even more a result of the ventilation/perfusion mismatch than the decrease in diffusing capacity. Even though the PaO_2 is reduced as a result of aging, in the absence of disease states the PaO_2 is adequate in providing for tissue oxygenation. Oxygen consumption declines with age in both males and females, which is partly due to decreased metabolism and the replacement of lean tissue with fat (Slonim and Hamilton, 1987).

CARBON DIOXIDE

Every aerobic metabolizing cell consumes oxygen and produces carbon dioxide. The carbon dioxide produced is continually eliminated from the body by pulmonary ventilation. While some **hypercapnia**—an elevated $PaCO_2$—is occasionally noted in elderly patients, there does not seem to be a consistent age-related alteration in the arterial partial pressure of carbon dioxide ($PaCO_2$). This could be a result of the greater diffusibility of carbon dioxide through the alveolar-capillary membrane and the differences in the oxygen and carbon dioxide dissociation curves (Levitzky, 1991).

CONTROL OF BREATHING

Older people do not increase their respiratory rates in response to lower levels of oxygen in the blood to the extent that they did when they were younger (Lamy, 1980). The ventilatory response to **hypoxemia**—low PaO_2—and resultant **hypoxia**—low oxygen at the tissue level—has been shown to decrease with age. Hypercapnia, when present, also elicits less of a ventilatory response in the elderly. These decreased responses could be the result of decreased sensitivity of the central and peripheral chemoreceptors. What is more likely, however, is that the previously mentioned changes in respiratory muscle strength, loss of elasticity, and lung and chest wall mechanics are the causative factors of a reduced ventilatory response in the aged.

IMPLICATIONS

There are a number of conclusions that can be drawn from this discussion of the aging body, and there are a number of implications for the respiratory care practitioner as well. Aging processes are normal, inevitable, and irreversible. Preservation of function, generally through exercise and good nutrition, is the best practice relative to the physiology of aging. Even those in their ninth decade of life respond well to moderate exercise and weight-lifting programs (Sobol and Fleming, 1994). Changes that naturally occur in the body as it ages may complicate treatment of the aged, or even mimic disease. For instance, an increased anterior-posterior diameter of the chest is normal in later life. Chop (1995) notes that this is because of an increased functional residual capacity (FRC). It should not be confused, however, with the barrel chest often seen with chronic obstructive pulmonary disease. Other changes in the upper body may complicate this differentiation. The shape of the chest is inevitably altered by the development of the so-called dowager's hump in older women, which is often the result of osteoporosis (Robinson, Weigley, and Mueller, 1993).

The most common symptom of respiratory distress in later life is dyspnea (Chop, 1995). Almost half of those age 70 and older have occasional exertional dyspnea. Nocturnal dyspnea and orthopnea usually indicate a cardiac cause underlying breathlessness, and denial of dyspnea is more common among older people with cardiovascular disease than among those with a respiratory disorder. Chest pain, however, is not always associated with myocardial ischemia. It can also be a sign of pneumonia, pulmonary emboli, pulmonary hypertension, muscle fatigue after severe coughing, or rib fracture, which is common among elderly people. Older people, especially those in long-term-care facilities, are also at a higher risk for infection with tuberculosis.

Pulmonary problems are among the most common postoperative complications among the aged (Sobol and Fleming, 1994). Older people with pneumonia may not cough, have a fever, or even an elevated white count. Confusion and functional deterioration may be the only signs of illness. Sobol and Fleming state that tachypnea and tachycardia with a change in functional status may be among the few signs present among older patients (1994).

Unfortunately, many older people with COPD are not aware of their disease until it reaches severe stages. Smoking is probably the single most important factor in the development of chronic obstructive pulmonary disease. "Clinical assessment of the elderly COPD patient includes a complete history and physical examination, as well as pre- and postbronchodilator spirometry to observe for bronchodilator response. A room-air arterial blood gas or pulse oximetry should be obtained to assess adequacy of oxygenation and possible need for oxygen therapy" (Sobol and Fleming, 1994, p. 42).

Most of the lung changes associated with aging are the result of the loss of elastic recoil of lung tissue and more collapsible airways. Lung volume and air flow rates change with aging. Because of the lost elastic recoil and gas trapping associated with airway collapse, residual volume increases. Pulmonary capacity declines among most very old people, which makes them increasingly vulnerable to respiratory distress and disease (Figure 3-3).

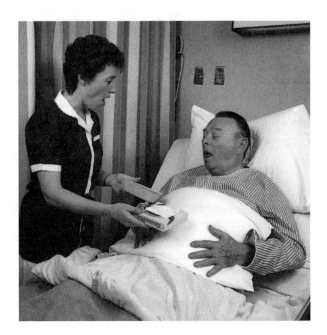

Figure 3-3 *Pulmonary capacity has declined among most older people.*

SUMMARY

COPD, pneumonia, influenza, and lung cancer account for about 15 percent of all deaths. These deaths, by their nature, are chronic—they take place over time and are characterized by increasing debility. No doubt many of them are preventable.

Age-related changes in the pulmonary system are predictable and measurable. In the presence of pulmonary disease, physiological alterations can result in crippling chronic conditions. Lack of disease and frequent exercise can delay some of these decremental changes. Elevated physical activity over a lifetime slows the rate of lung-chest degeneration (Martin and Youtsey, 1988).

Review Questions

1. What evidence have you seen among older people that would support the basic wear and tear theory of aging?
2. What do you think would be the most difficult part of pulmonary function testing among older patients?
3. What theory of aging accounts for the fact that meat from old animals is tougher than meat from younger animals?
4. Explain the genetic basis of the biological time clock.

5. What happens with loss of elastic recoil of lung tissue?
6. What chronic pulmonary conditions among the aged are most preventable?
7. How are the autoimmune and free radical theories of aging related?
8. What is the effect of osteoporosis on the breathing capacity of older women?
9. Why would older people consider functional capacity to be more important than disease condition when assessing their own health?

References

Carrel, A., and Burrows, M. T. (1911). On the physiochemical regulation of the growth of tissues. *Journal of Experimental Medicine, 13,* 562–570.

Centers for Disease Control (1995, January 31). *Monthly Vital Statistics Report, 43* (8).

Centers for Disease Control (1996, October 4). *Monthly Vital Statistics Report, 45* (3), supplement 2.

Chalker, R. B., and Celli, B. R. (1993). Special considerations in the elderly patient. *Clinics in Chest Medicine, 14,* 437–442.

Chop, W. C. (1995). Resources for an aging population. *RT—The Journal for Respiratory Care Practitioners, 8* (11), 25–30.

Des Jardins, T. (1993). *Cardiopulmonary anatomy and physiology: Essentials for respiratory care.* Albany, NY: Delmar.

Harman, D. (1968). Free radical theory of aging: Effect of free radical reaction inhibitors in the mortality rate of male LAF mice. *Journal of Gerontology, 23,* 476–490.

Hayflick, L. (1974). The strategy of senescence. *The Gerontologist, 14,* 37–45.

Lamy, P. P. (1980). *Prescribing for the elderly.* New York: PSG Publishing.

Levitzky, M. G. (1991). *Pulmonary physiology,* 3rd ed. New York: McGraw-Hill.

Levitzky, M. G., Cairo, J. M., and Hall, S. M. (1990). *Introduction to respiratory care.* Philadelphia: W. B. Saunders.

Lough, M. O., Doershuk, C. F., and Stern, R. C. (1985). *Pediatric respiratory therapy.* Chicago: Yearbook Medical Publishers.

Makinodan, T. (1977). Immunity and aging. In C. Finch and L. Hayflick (Eds.), *Handbook of the biology of aging.* New York: Van Nostrand Reinhold, pp. 379–408.

Martin, D. E., and Youtsey, J. (1988). *Respiratory anatomy and physiology.* St. Louis, MO: C. V. Mosby.

Masoro, E. J., Katz, M. S., and McMahan, C. A. (1989). Evidence for the glycation hypothesis of aging from the food-restricted rodent model. *Journal of Gerontology: Biological Sciences, 44,* B20–22.

McCay, C., Crowell, M., and Maynard, L. (1935). The effect of retarded growth upon the length of life and upon ultimate size. *Journal of Nutrition, 10,* 63–79.

Miller, J., and Keane, C. (1992). *Encyclopedia and dictionary of medicine, nursing, and allied health.* Philadelphia: W. B. Saunders.

Murray, J. F. (1986). *The normal lung.* Philadelphia: W. B. Saunders.

Ranga, V., Kleinerman, J., and Sorensen, J. (1979). Age-related changes in elastic fibers and elastin of lung. *American Review of Respiratory Disease, 119,* 369–375.

Robinson, C. H., Weigley, E. S., and Mueller, D. H. (1993). *Basic nutrition and diet therapy.* New York: Macmillan.

Shock, N. (1976). The physiology of aging. In *Human physiology and the environment.* San Francisco: W. H. Freeman.

Slonim, N. B., and Hamilton, L. H. (1987). *Respiratory physiology.* St. Louis, MO: C. V. Mosby.

Sobol, E., and Fleming, R. (1994). Treating the aged. *Advance for Managers of Respiratory Care, 3* (10), 41–43.

Spence, A. P. (1989). *Biology of human aging.* Englewood Cliffs, NJ: Prentice-Hall.

Thorson, J. A. (1995). *Aging in a changing society.* Belmont, CA: Wadsworth.

Tierney, L. M., McPhee, S. J., and Papadakis, M. A. (1995). *Current medical diagnosis and treatment 1995.* Norwalk, CT: Appleton & Lange.

CHAPTER FOUR

CHRONIC DISEASES OF THE ELDERLY

KEY TERMS

agammaglobulinemia
alpha$_1$ antiprotease
aneurysm
ascites
athersclerosis
arteriosclerosis
atopic
backward failure
carcinogens
cerebrovascular
   accident (CVA)
Charcot-Brouchard
   aneurysm

Cheyne-Stokes
   breathing
cor pulmonale
dyskinesia
elastase
granulomas
hemiplegia
hemoptysis
hemorrhage
homeostenosis
ideopathic
intima

ischemia
ischemic heart disease
kyphoscoliosis
kyphosis
neoplasms
orthopnea
paroxysmal nocturnal
   dyspnea
polycythemia
septum
thrombus

LEARNING OBJECTIVES

After completing this chapter, the reader should be able to:

1. Identify the leading causes of mortality from chronic disease in the elderly.
2. Differentiate between coronary artery disease and congestive heart failure.
3. List possible interventions to decrease the risk of heart disease.
4. Define stroke and explain why the diagnosis, treatment, and prevention of stroke are important to health care professionals.

5. Compare and contrast the causes and consequences of chronic obstructive pulmonary disease.
6. Explain the differences between old lungs and emphysematous lungs.
7. Compare and contrast the causes and consequences of chronic restrictive pulmonary disease.
8. Describe the role of rehabilitation programs in the management of chronic cardiopulmonary diseases.
9. Define cancer and describe predisposing factors, symptoms, treatment, and prevention of lung cancer.
10. Identify factors that place the elderly at risk for developing tuberculosis.

INTRODUCTION

Age-related changes in the body's defense mechanisms and the biological aging process lead to gradual decremental changes in the functional capacity of most of the body's systems. These decremental changes are referred to as homeostenosis (Tierney et al., 1995). Changes begin when adults are in their thirties and continue in a gradual and linear downward slope. The rate of decline in each organ system is variable and dependent on environmental factors, diet, heredity, habits, and disease. This chapter highlights the more common chronic diseases associated with aging that have an effect on the cardiopulmonary system.

Chronic, derived from the Greek term *chronikos*, implies a disease of long duration. Chronic diseases are often the result of the decline in organ systems, regardless of whether the cause is extrinsic or intrinsic. Chronic implies that the condition has persisted for a reasonable length of time and shows little change or extremely slow change over time. People who are chronologically and biologically older are the most likely ones to have chronic diseases. However, younger people are by no means eliminated from having chronic illness.

By the time people reach age 65 and older, the top six causes of death are chronic illnesses (Thorson, 1995):

1. Heart disease
2. Cancer
3. Stroke
4. Chronic obstructive pulmonary disease
5. Pneumonia/influenza
6. Diabetes

Chronic diseases of the cardiac and pulmonary systems account for a major proportion of the deaths in later life. This should not, however, be interpreted to mean that all chronic illnesses result in death. Most older people have at least one chronic condition and many have multiple chronic illnesses. The majority of older people cope with these slowly progressing illnesses over a period of many years (Figure 4-1). In many cases, the diseases do not restrict their ability to perform the activities of daily living until near the end of life. The focus of this chapter is on the cardiopulmonary chronic illnesses. Other chronic conditions more prevalent among the elderly are briefly summarized.

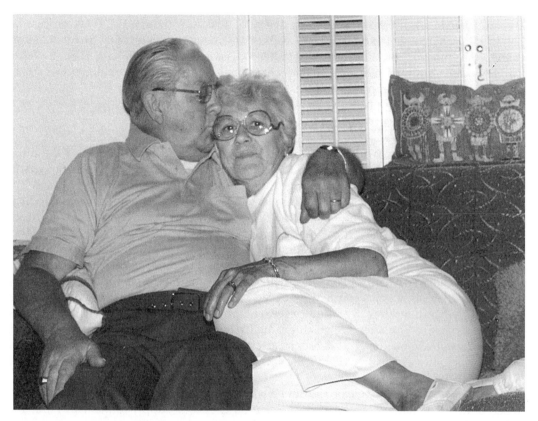

Figure 4-1 *Chronic conditions such as diabetes, congestive heart failure, arthritis, and cataracts do not prevent this couple from leading an independent life style.*

HEART DISEASE

Heart disease includes disorders of the heart and vascular system. It implies that there is a heart abnormality or failure to function properly.

Reviewing the physiological changes in the aging heart sets the stage for discussing chronic heart disease. As with other muscles, the cardiac muscle develops increasing amounts of collagen and fat with advanced age (Hogstel, 1994). Considering the amount of work done by the heart over the course of a lifetime, certain other anatomical changes are to be expected (Marieb, 1992). There is a gradual sclerosis and thickening of the heart valves. The mitral valve, due to the increased workload of the left ventricle, becomes less efficient. There is a decline in cardiac reserve. A blunted response to stress, a reduction in sympathetic control of the heart, and a gradual increase in the variability of the heart rate may also be noted. Fibrosis of the cardiac muscle and conduction system can lead to arrhythmias. The vascular system may show atherosclerotic changes that can result in hypertensive heart disease and coronary artery occlusion. Although the aging process it-self leads to changes in the blood vessel walls, many investigators feel that diet, not aging, is the single most important contributor to heart disease (Marieb, 1992).

Heart disease is the leading cause of death in the United States. Therefore, much atten-tion is focused on its prevention and treatment.

CORONARY ARTERY DISEASE

Coronary artery disease, which is also referred to as **ischemic heart disease,** is the most widespread form of heart disease. Coronary artery disease is a condition in which there is an obstruction or progressive narrowing of the coronary arteries, the ones that feed the heart itself. Obstruction in the interior lumen of the blood vessels will ultimately reduce blood flow. **Ischemia** is an inadequate blood flow to any part of the body. Ischemic heart disease is reduced blood flow through the coronary arteries that supply oxygenated blood to the myocardium. The end result is an insufficient oxygen supply (Dantzker et al., 1995).

Although all of the factors leading to the narrowing of the coronary arteries are not completely known, two major contributing factors are **atherosclerosis** and **arteriosclero-sis.** Atherosclerosis is the accumulation of fat, cholesterol, and fibrous connective tissue in the **intima,** the interior wall of the arteries. This buildup of accumulated substances pro-gressively narrows the arteries, which gradually but eventually leads to reduced blood flow. Although the incidence of coronary artery disease statistically correlates with age, some investigators have speculated that atherosclerosis is not necessarily age related (Barrow, 1989).

Coronary occlusion can also be associated with thrombosis, or clotting. Blood clots occur when undissolved fatty deposits in arteries cut off the blood supply to the heart, thus re-sulting in ischemia.

Arteriosclerosis, commonly associated with atherosclerosis, is actually a thickening and hardening of the walls of the arteries. Arteriosclerosis involves the **media,** the middle mus-cular layer of the arterial wall, as well as the intima. Arteriosclerosis results in the loss of elasticity of the arterial walls. Many researchers have concluded that, unlike atherosclero-sis, arteriosclerosis is clearly age related (Barrow, 1989). Commonly called hardening of the arteries, arteriosclerosis also narrows the lumen of the coronary arteries and results in a di-minished blood supply to the heart. Atherosclerosis and arteriosclerosis are both present in many elderly patients.

Coronary artery disease can develop very gradually. Many individuals in their thirties and forties already have some measure of the disease (Freiberg, 1992). As with any chronic condition, heart disease may be progressively debilitating.

When the degree of severity of obstruction advances from chronic to acute and causes damage to the heart muscle, symptoms such as shortness of breath, dizziness, confusion, and pain may be present.

Angina Pectoris.   Angina pectoris is acute chest pain that results from myocardial is-chemia. Angina pectoris, although not a disease entity, is precipitated by any underlying disease process involving vessels that supply blood and oxygen to the heart. Angina pec-toris can also be caused by aortic stenosis, pulmonary stenosis, and ventricular hypertrophy. Approximately 10 out of every 1,000 persons age 55 or older are believed to have angina pectoris (Reiss and Evans, 1993).

Treatment of Angina Pectoris. Coronary vasodilators are primarily used in the treatment of angina pectoris. The most commonly used pharmacological vasodilators are the nitrates, including nitroglycerine. There are two theories of how these agents reduce anginal pain. The first suggests that nitrates improve oxygen delivery by increasing coronary blood flow and redistributing perfusion to ischemic tissues. The second theory contends that nitrates reduce oxygen consumption by coronary blood vessels, thus relieving ischemia. Recent evidence seems to indicate that the latter theory is more likely to be accurate (Reiss and Evans, 1993). Nitroglycerine is available in many dosage forms. With all forms of nitroglycerine, dosages should be titrated in the elderly, based on the patient's response to it. During maintenance therapy, a nitrate-free period of approximately 10 to 12 hours per day should be provided, which will prevent tolerance development (Bloom and Schlom, 1993).

Some potential adverse effects that are of particular concern among older patients include rebound angina that may occur with abrupt nitrate withdrawal and common symptoms of hypotension, syncope, headache, and tachycardia. Older adults may also develop contact dermatitis when the paste or patch dosage form is utilized (Bloom and Schlom, 1993). Factors related to the development of atherosclerosis are easier to control than those of arteriosclerosis. Patients should be educated about their condition. Situations frequently resulting in angina should be identified and avoided, if possible. Smoking should be discouraged. In addition to the many health hazards associated with tobacco, nicotine is a vasoconstrictor and may counteract the effects of any vasodilator medication prescribed for the patient. Diets low in fat, cholesterol, and calories are recommended. Stress reduction has a vasodilating effect. A great deal of research has been done demonstrating that even severe heart disease can often be reversed with alterations in diet (Ornish, 1993). Nonpharmalogical interventions are viewed as an alternative therapeutic regimen for many patients with coronary artery disease.

CONGESTIVE HEART FAILURE

Congestive heart failure (CHF) encompasses a variety of conditions that lead to or result in a diminished pumping ability of the heart. CHF is one cause of decreased cardiac output. If decreased enough, the heart may be unable to provide adequate perfusion to meet the body's metabolic needs. The most common causes of CHF in the elderly are hypertension, cardiomyopathy, valvular disease, and ischemic heart disease (Needham, 1993). Congestive heart failure may be classified as either chronic or acute. It may be the result of either left ventricular failure, right ventricular failure, or both. Even though both left and right ventricular failure can precipitate CHF, there are a few distinguishing symptoms to differentiate them.

Left Ventricular Failure. Left ventricular failure seriously reduces systemic perfusion, which leaves patients feeling weak and tired. If pulmonary venous return exceeds the output of the left ventricle, the end result is increased pulmonary venous pressure, increased pulmonary capillary hydrostatic pressure, and eventual pulmonary vascular congestion. Symptoms secondary to pulmonary congestion are decreased compliance and stimulation of the J receptors in the interstitium, which results in dyspnea or rapid shallow breathing.

In CHF, dyspnea on exertion may be the first symptom noted. Gradually, dyspnea may extend to the resting hours and be manifested as **paroxysmal nocturnal dyspnea.** Patients may also experience **orthopnea,** more dyspnea in a recumbent position and less dyspnea when they are in an upright or semi-Fowler's position. When the cardiac output becomes more compromised and blood flow to the brain is reduced, other symptoms such as behavioral changes, poor memory, irritability, and restlessness may ensue (Hogstel, 1994).

Another characteristic of left-sided failure in some patients is an abnormal ventilatory pattern called **Cheyne-Stokes breathing.** Cheyne-Stokes is a cyclical breathing pattern in which gradually increasing tidal volumes are followed by gradually decreasing tidal volumes separated by periods of apnea. In the case of left-sided congestive heart failure, it has generally been proposed that prolonged circulation time delays normal transmission of messages from the chemoreceptors to the brain. Reduced systemic perfusion thus results in an abnormal delay between the events in the lungs and chemoreceptor sensing of PaO_2/$PaCO_2$ changes. These transmission delays result in the oscillating Cheyne-Stokes pattern (Weinberger, 1986; Dantzker, MacIntyre, and Bakow, 1995).

Right Ventricular Failure. Right ventricular failure, leading to congestive heart failure is similar to left ventricular failure in that both are pump problems. The distinguishing symptoms vary, depending on which ventricle the fluid accumulates behind. Right ventricle failure is most commonly caused by left ventricular failure (Dantzker, MacIntyre, and Bakow, 1995). The ventricles share a common wall, the **septum,** which is affected by, and contributes to failure of, the other side. It is also possible for left-sided failure to cause right-sided failure by increasing pressures in pulmonary circulation. This is known as **backward failure** (Levitzky, Cairo, and Hall, 1990).

Other causes of right ventricular failure involve an acute or chronic pressure overload of the right ventricle. Mitral stenosis and pulmonary valve stenosis can cause elevated left atrial pressure, which in turn can result in pulmonary hypertension.

Pulmonary Diseases. Pulmonary diseases themselves can also produce pulmonary hypertension, which eventually puts the pressure overload directly back on the right ventricle. Pulmonary emboli that occlude the vessels, and hypoxia, which causes vasoconstriction, are both contributors to elevated pulmonary vascular pressures. When pulmonary hypertension is due to disorders of the pulmonary parenchyma or pulmonary vessels, the resulting right ventricular hypertrophy is known as **cor pulmonale.** Many patients seen by respiratory care practitioners have some measure of right ventricular hypertrophy. Chronic hypoxia, caused by a variety of pulmonary disorders, results in production of more red blood cells by the bone marrow. Increased levels of red blood cells, known as **polycythemia,** increase the viscosity of the blood. In some pulmonary diseases, such as emphysema, there is destruction not only of alveolar tissue but also of the capillary bed surrounding the alveoli. Chronic hypoxia-induced vasoconstriction, increased blood viscosity, and a reduction of functioning capillary bed contribute to the development of cor pulmonale.

The main sign of right ventricular failure, whether precipitated by cardiac valvular problems or pulmonary vascular problems, is venous congestion (Levitzky, Cairo, and Hall, 1990). The accumulation of venous blood in the large veins may be noted clinically as distended neck veins. Chronic venous congestion of the liver may lead to liver dysfunction and cirrhosis. Elevated venous pressure eventually causes back pressure on the capillaries, resulting in a net filtration of fluid out of the capillaries. As edema fluid is produced, it tends to collect in gravity-dependent regions, causing swelling of the ankles and feet. Bilateral, dependent, pitting edema is commonly seen in patients with congestive heart failure and cor pulmonale. Peripheral edema, venous congestion, pulmonary vascular congestion, and even fluid retention secondary to impaired renal perfusion are associated with congestive heart failure.

Treatment.   Treatment of CHF is multifaceted, just as are its precipitating causes. Increasing cardiac output will increase tissue perfusion and relieve pulmonary and systemic vascular congestion. Cardiac glycosides usually provide effective treatment, since they increase the force of myocardial contractions (Reiss and Evans, 1993), thereby increasing cardiac output. Unfortunately, some glycosides, Digoxin being the most popular in the United States, have a very narrow therapeutic range. The elderly are more likely to develop digoxin toxicity, which may cause arrhythmias (Bloom and Schlom, 1993).

Oxygen therapy is very important in treating CHF. Correction of alveolar hypoxia and hypoxemia, and maintaining a PaO_2 at a level greater than 60 torr, will help eliminate hypoxic vasoconstriction. Diuretics and low-sodium diets may be beneficial in some patients. When congestive heart failure is secondary to other factors, it is best to correct the underlying problem. In all cases, treatment is directed at controlling the heart failure (Needham, 1993).

There are other less frequently diagnosed cardiac problems in the elderly, such as cardiomyopathies, pericardial abnormalities, and valvular dysfunction. Any damage or compromise to the cardiovascular system increases the risk for mortality. The various forms of arteriosclerosis, atherosclerosis, and resultant hypertension cause a high percentage of heart attacks and strokes. Added together, heart attacks and strokes are the most common causes of death in the United States.

CEREBROVASCULAR DISEASE

Cerebrovascular disease includes the disorders of the vessels of the cerebrum—the brain. Cerebrovascular disease is another leading cause of death in North America. The most common nervous system disorder, a degenerative disease of the central nervous system, is **cerebrovascular accident (CVA)** or stroke.

What may be of more significance to health care providers than the mortality rate from strokes, however, is the number of older people disabled by strokes. As indicated in Chapter 2, stroke is also the underlying cause of multi-infarct dementia. Thus, CVA is often the precipitating event for a great deal of the physical and psychological disability among the aged. Stroke is one of the most frequent causes of long-term-care institutionalization

(Thorson, 1995). As therapists move into subacute care employment, understanding the etiology as well as the warning signs and prevention of stroke takes on new importance.

STROKES

Strokes are caused by an interruption of blood flow through one or more blood vessels of the brain. Elderly individuals are at risk for stroke syndrome due to the increased incidence of hypertension, atherosclerosis, and heart disease in later life. Smoking, obesity, and diabetes are also risk factors for stroke. Strokes are the third leading cause of death for persons age 65 and older, after heart disease and cancer.

There are three primary causes of strokes: cerebral thrombosis, cerebral embolism, and cerebral hemorrhage. They are all related to the pathological condition of the vascular system and are associated with an infarct in the brain tissue.

Cerebral Thrombosis.   A cerebral blood clot, or **thrombus,** is the most common cause of stroke. Atherosclerosis is the main culprit, leading to narrowing of the vascular lumen. A thrombus—an aggregation of platelets, fibrin, and cellular elements—can form whenever the flow of blood is impeded. Thrombosis may produce edema and ischemia of the surrounding brain tissue. This cause of stroke usually has a gradual onset of symptoms.

Cerebral Embolism.   Cerebral embolism is the result of a small mass, perhaps an air bubble, a fat globule, a piece of tissue, or a thrombus, that settles in a vessel and causes a blockage. Embolic strokes are characterized by a sudden onset, as the interruption to blood flow happens quickly. Cerebral embolism is the second most common cause of stroke. Strokes resulting from an embolus may occur at any age, but are more common among people with some history of cardiac disease (Hamann, 1994). Embolic strokes are often associated with a recent heart attack, a dysfunctional valve, recent valve replacement surgery, or even atrial fibrillation (Freiberg, 1992).

Cerebral Hemorrhage.   The third type of stroke is caused by a **hemorrhage,** or a rupturing of a blood vessel within the brain. Hemorrhage may occur at any age; among younger persons it may be the result of a congenital abnormality. A weak spot in a blood vessel in the brain, which existed at birth, may finally rupture. Strokes as a result of cerebral hemorrhages are more common after age 50, however, probably as a result of hypertension. Blood vessels weakened by arteriosclerosis may not be able to withstand higher systemic pressures over a long period of time. An **aneurysm,** or balloonlike dilation of an artery, may also be the result of damaged or weakened arterial walls. In the presence of hypertension, aneurysms may be more susceptible to rupture and may cause hemorrhage into the brain tissue. A **Charcot-Brouchard aneurysm** is a small aneurysm found on a tiny artery in the cerebral cortex or basal ganglia (Stedman, 1994). Charcot-Brouchard occurs more frequently in older hypertensive individuals. These aneurysms may rupture, causing massive cerebral hemorrhage.

Hemorrhagic strokes occur most often during the day while the person is active. Strokes caused by cerebral hemorrhage usually produce more extensive neurologic defects, resulting in slower recovery than strokes from other causes. As a general rule, those who become unconscious from a stroke have a poorer prognosis of recovery. The length of time of unconsciousness and a poorer prognosis of recovery are related in a direct linear fashion. A person who is unconscious for 24 hours or more after a stroke has a very poor prognosis, particularly in comparison to someone who was unconscious for only a few minutes. There are different forms of strokes based on their course of progress.

Transient Ischemic Attack.   Transient ischemic attack (TIA) is not uncommon in older adults. TIA is a "little" stroke that may last anywhere from seconds to hours. A transient ischemic attack is a mild form of obstruction to the blood flow in the cerebral vessels that may be caused by a blockage or simply a spasmlike narrowing of one of the vessels. It may result in fainting and may be a precursor to a major stroke. In some cases the TIA is so fleeting that it is almost unrecognizable.

CASE STUDY

It had been an exciting day. Peter was graduating from high school. Grandpa Pete, age 83, was joining in the celebration. He had traveled with his daughter and son-in-law from Oklahoma for the occasion. Up until 4 years previously, Grandpa Pete had been relatively healthy and active enough to play an occasional round of golf. In recent years, though, a heart attack, a fractured hip, and Alzheimer's disease had taken its toll. Still enjoying mealtime and family activities, however, Grandpa Pete joined in the dinner table chatter. While the family discussed plans for the graduation it became evident that Grandpa had stopped eating and talking. Slightly slumped over in his wheelchair and gazing into space, his silence frightened everyone. His daughter, who was a nurse, quickly reassured the family: "Don't be afraid. Grandpa just had a TIA." Not knowing what a TIA was, everyone was terrified. She placed Grandpa on the couch, put him in a half-sitting, half-reclining position, and secured him with pillows. Within minutes, Grandpa had regained full consciousness but was very confused and disoriented. He wasn't able to go to the graduation ceremony that evening, but he did recover fully from the TIA.

Symptoms that may accompany this brief neurologic deficit include dizziness, slurred speech, uncoordinated walking, weakness or numbness to one side of the body, and double vision. Seizure activity may also be noted post-TIA. As the name implies, the symptoms are transient and reversible. When recognized as an early warning sign of an impending stroke, some intervention may be possible. The majority of people who experience a TIA can be treated successfully, and most can be prevented from experiencing a major stroke (Hogstel, 1994). TIAs should not be ignored. Although the symptoms are temporary, transient ischemic attacks are red flags that warn of more serious CVAs (Marieb, 1992).

Stroke in Evolution.   A progressive stroke, or stroke in evolution (SIE), may begin with a slight neurologic impairment and gradually worsen over a period of a few days (Hamann, 1994). Symptoms may include a gradual but progressive weakness on one side of the body.

Completed Stroke. In a completed stroke (CS) the damage is maximal in the beginning. Patients with a completed stroke exhibit symptoms associated with severe cerebral ischemia. The symptoms occur suddenly, with possible unconsciousness, heavy breathing caused by paralysis of a portion of the soft palate, and unequal pupil size. Paralysis is directly related to the area of cerebral ischemia. Damage to the left side of the brain often leads to paralysis of the face, arm, and leg on the right side, and vice versa. Completed strokes, while rarely causing sudden death, are much more serious than TIAs and usually result in permanent paralysis and sensory deficits. Fewer than 35 percent of those surviving an initial CVA are alive 3 years later. Patients suffering CVAs from blood clots are likely to have recurrent clotting problems and additional strokes (Marieb, 1992).

Prevention. Prevention of stroke is by far more preferable than is treatment. Prevention depends on controlling or eliminating risk factors as much as possible. Diet and exercise, aimed at reducing hypertension and atherosclerosis, are primary. Medical management of preexisting chronic conditions, which may include hypertension, obesity, diabetes, and heart disease, also reduce the incidence of stroke. Health care workers need to be cognizant of CVA warning signs. Prompt medical attention may help to prevent disabling strokes.

Treatment. Treatment varies, depending on the reason for the stroke. If the cause of the stroke is embolic and hemorrhage has been ruled out, anticoagulants may be used. Antihypertensive agents are helpful in reducing blood pressure within the vessel and avoiding rupture. Long-acting angiotensin-converting enzyme (ACE) inhibitors have been found safe and effective in treating hypertension in the elderly (Hawkins, Hall, and Douglas, 1994). A surgical procedure, carotid endarterectomy, may be performed to surgically remove clots that have lodged in the carotid or vertebral arteries in the neck. Recent research suggests that carotid endarterectomy can be performed in an elderly population with morbidity and mortality rates similar to those of a much younger population (Coyle et al., 1994).

Rehabilitation. Rehabilitation for stroke patients is successful in varying degrees depending on the severity of the stroke. The obvious goal is to return the patient to a state as near to normal as possible.

Respiratory care practitioners are increasingly finding employment in settings such as rehabilitation hospitals, subacute care facilities, and skilled nursing facilities. They find themselves working with speech, physical, and occupational therapists, as well as nurses and dietitians, to effect positive outcomes in elderly stroke patients (Figure 4-2).

For some older patients, palliative care may replace rehabilitative efforts. When a return to functional status is not the goal, then care must focus on comfort and prevention of further complications. Airway patency and adequate oxygenation maintenance is critical. Suctioning may be necessary if paralysis interferes with normal airway clearance mechanisms. Frequent turning is needed to prevent pressure necrosis. Nutritional needs must be addressed and accomplished by whatever means are necessary. Prevention of aspiration is also critical. Stroke victims often have an impaired swallowing response and are likely to choke.

Some elderly patients revert to mouth breathing, which dries the oral mucosal membrane. There is an age-associated loss of water in the epidural layer and a thinning of the

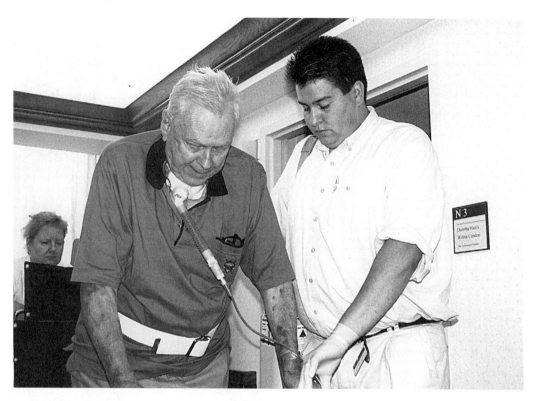

Figure 4-2 *Poststroke respiratory patient with a therapist doing gait training.*

mucosal epidermis. Elderly patients may be at risk for oral skin breakdown and infection. Gentle cleansing of the mouth on a regular basis is recommended (Figure 4-3). Rinsing the mouth with a nonalcohol-based mouthwash may be helpful. Soft toothbrushes and toothettes may also be used to cleanse the mouth. Overuse of lemon-glycerine swabs is not recommended as glycerine is drying to mouth tissues (Needham, 1993).

Knowledge of chronic disease processes and intervention strategies is becoming more important all the time. Many comorbid conditions can be found in patients with chronic pulmonary disease. The emphasis of elder care is to treat the whole patient, not just each particular problem or disease. Respiratory care personnel should take advantage of educational programs that focus or provide information on the total geriatric patient care continuum.

CHRONIC OBSTRUCTIVE PULMONARY DISEASE

Management of chronic pulmonary disease in the elderly would appear to be the obvious focus of this chapter. In actuality, most readers of this text should already be well versed in pulmonary disease management. Without going into a great deal of repetitive detail, this

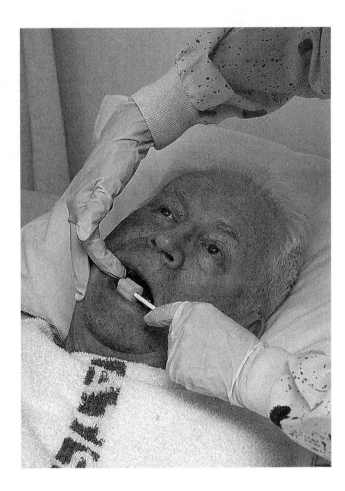

Figure 4-3 *Oral care being administered to an elderly patient.*

section focuses more on age-related consequences and how they predispose patients to lung disease.

Growth and development of the respiratory system usually ceases somewhere in the twenties. Most people demonstrate peak performance on their pulmonary function tests (PFTs) between the ages of 20 and 25, after which there is a slow, progressive decline (Levitzky, Cairo, and Hall, 1990). Chapter 3 outlines many of the physiological age-related changes that functionally affect the lungs. The loss of elastic recoil, loss of alveolar surface area, increased residual volume, increased air trapping, decreased support of small airways, and decreased respiratory muscle strength could all be describing emphysema.

Chronic disease is a major threat to the independence of older people. Usually, chronic diseases do not occur independently. Instead, they are multiple in nature (Giordano, 1993). Chronic obstructive pulmonary disease (COPD) is a good example. COPD is a leading cause of morbidity and functional disability among older adults. Chronic bronchitis and emphysema are both more common among older people. These two diseases, although diagnostically different, may occur together.

EMPHYSEMA

Emphysema is distinguished from chronic bronchitis and asthma by an abnormal anatomy of the terminal airways that shows destruction or loss of alveolar or respiratory bronchioles, or both (Witek and Schachter, 1994). In emphysema, the bronchioles and alveolar walls are destroyed as a result of an imbalance between **elastase,** a lung protease that breaks down elastin, and **alpha₁ antiprotease,** an antielastase substance (Figure 4-4). This destruction interferes with both the mechanics of breathing and gas exchange. Emphysema is sometimes subdivided into four different types—centrilobular, panlobular, paraseptal, and irregular—according to the anatomical location in one or both lungs (Hamann, 1994; Levitzky, Cairo, and Hall, 1990). When treating the emphysema patient at bedside, type designation is usually inconsequential.

In contrast to the diagnosis of chronic bronchitis, which is largely based on clinical presentation, emphysema is formally a pathologic diagnosis (Weinberger, 1986). Although lung biopsies are rarely done for diagnostic purposes, there may be postmortem confirmation of emphysema. Surveys from England, Canada, and Sweden show that emphysema is rare in persons under the age of 30, but that its prevalence increases quickly in patients over the age of 50 (Witek and Schachter, 1994). Up to 65 percent of men and 15 percent of women examined by autopsy showed some evidence of emphysema (Witek and Schachter, 1994).

Currently, two major factors have been identified as causative agents in pulmonary emphysema: cigarette smoking and a hereditary factor known as alpha₁ antiprotease deficiency. Genetic factors are responsible for a very small percentage of patients diagnosed with emphysema. Cigarette smoking is the underlying cause for most cases, although the exact mechanism is still poorly understood. Researchers and theorists speculate that the normal balance of elastase/antielastase enzymes is somehow altered by smoking. Whether

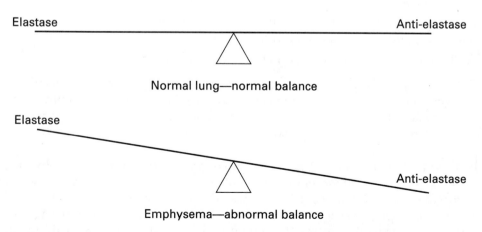

Figure 4-4 *Abnormal elastase balance.*

smoking triggers an increased production of elastase or inhibits the production of antielastase, the end result is the same. There is destruction of alveolar tissue (Farzan, 1992). There are, of course, nonsmokers with nongenetic emphysema and smokers who have no trace of the disease.

Although the symptoms and functional abnormalities of old lungs and emphysematous lungs may be similar, it is important to note that there are differences. Possible age-related loss of elastin—along with overdistention and hyperinflation of the old lungs due to loss of elastic recoil—is not the same as the destructive alveolar changes noted with emphysema (Farzan, 1992). Unfortunately, many older adults suffer from both problems.

CHRONIC BRONCHITIS

Chronic bronchitis, also classified as a chronic obstructive pulmonary disease, is characterized by excessive mucus production. Clinically, the diagnosis is made when the patient has a productive cough for at least 3 consecutive months, for 2 successive years.

Two major factors associated with chronic bronchitis are tobacco smoking and age. Many patients with chronic bronchitis are accustomed to their morning cough and excess sputum production. Because it does not noticeably interfere with their lives, they feel no need to seek medical care. Many individuals have no symptoms until middle age. Dyspnea on exertion may be the first indication that there is a problem. Because the dyspnea is usually mild at first, many people will simply adjust their level of activity to avoid this symptom. Dyspnea is not normal nor is it age related. When dyspnea becomes pronounced as a result of severe airway obstruction, the patient is diagnosed as having chronic obstructive bronchitis.

By far the most important etiologic agent in the development of chronic bronchitis is cigarette smoking. There are five notable pathological changes that occur as a result of chronic exposure to smoke (Martin, 1988):

- Depression of ciliary movement
- Loss of ciliated epithelium
- Replacement of ciliated epithelium by flat squamous cells
- Increased mucus production by existing goblet cells
- Appearance of more goblet cells and thus more mucus

Elderly individuals already have a diminished mucociliary clearance mechanism. Airway obstruction as a result of accumulated secretions due to smoking can turn a chronic disease into an acute exacerbation. The exacerbation then becomes an acute respiratory emergency requiring medical attention.

Treatment and Prevention.   To a large degree, chronic bronchitis and emphysema are preventable. In light of all recent evidence linking smoking to chronic lung disease, the most effective preventive measure against these diseases is smoking cessation.

A very important phase in the treatment of COPD involves outpatient management or home therapy. Technical advances of respiratory support have extended the lives of many with chronic diseases (Lucas et al., 1988).

COPD in its later stages leads to chronic hypoxemia. Data from numerous multicenter studies have led to one conclusion: Correction of hypoxemia is the single most important therapy to improve survival of patients with COPD (O'Donohue, 1988). Oxygen therapy prolongs lives (Figure 4-5). To date, there is no definitive evidence that other forms of therapy such as bronchodilators or corticosteroids prolong survival. Despite the proven efficacy and numerous benefits of long-term oxygen therapy in patients with COPD, the cost remains substantial. The annual expenditures involved in supplying home oxygen therapy to patients in the United States exceeded the entire budget of the National Heart, Lung, and Blood Institute in 1993, a sum equal to $1.1 billion (O'Donohue and Plummer, 1995).

Management of COPD at home also involves education for both patients and their families. Home care and medical supply companies offer a variety of services, types of equipment, and supplies to patients at home. There are many effective drugs on the market that have been proven to relieve the symptoms of airway obstruction. Patient comprehension, however, must precede patient compliance. This is imperative if these therapeutic modalities are to be successful. Patient cooperation and compliance with the prescribed treatment usually depends on their understanding of their disease and measures directed toward it (Farzan, 1992).

Older patients provide special challenges for home care providers. As Americans age, an increasing percentage of people are living into their eighties, nineties, and beyond. It is

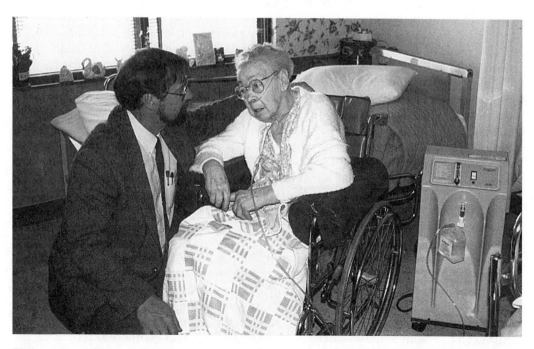

Figure 4-5 *Oxygen is provided via a concentrator to an elderly COPD (chronic obstructive pulmonary disease) patient in a nursing home.*

among these age groups that personal care and support from both families and health providers is needed (Haddad, 1987). In describing those 85 and older, many of whom have COPD, it would be unfair and inaccurate to assume that all are alike. They tend, however, to have a greater likelihood as a group to have thinner bones, weaker muscles, poorer eyesight and hearing, slower responses, and more compromised immune systems. Most have multiple chronic problems, regularly use multiple prescription medications, have modest memory loss, and often have problems with mobility.

Home care providers need to be increasingly creative in devising ways to successfully allow patients the maximum benefits of therapy. Because frail elderly people do not respond well to hospitalization, the goal must be to keep them home as long as possible.

In addition to the general pharmacological and therapeutic regimens followed by older individuals with COPD, another preventive strategy needs to be mentioned. Vaccines against specific strains of influenza and pneumonia are available. Older adults with compromised immune systems are not as likely to be successfully immunized as are younger adults receiving the same serum, but any protection is better than none.

CHRONIC ASTHMA

Asthma is found in a substantial number of geriatric patients. It is estimated that between 3 and 10 percent of the general population of the United States falls into the clinical diagnostic category of asthma (Hazzard et al., 1994; Witek and Schachter, 1994). Although more than half of these asthmatics develop the disease before their early teens, it is estimated that 10 percent of asthmatics develop the disease after age 65 (Witek and Schachter, 1994). A fairly recent publication of the American Lung Association (1993) states that more than 10 million people have asthma, and almost 1.1 million of those people are 65 or older.

Research and knowledge of this disease have somewhat changed the definition of asthma over recent years. Currently, the accepted definition is as follows: "Asthma is characterized by airway inflammation, airway obstruction that is usually reversible, and increased airway responsiveness to a variety of stimuli" (*JACI*, 1991).

The underdiagnosis of asthma appears to be common, especially in older adults (Hazzard et al., 1994). Diagnosis of asthma in geriatric patients is occasionally missed. Asthma in the aged is likely to be called COPD (Kyes, 1994). According to Benjamin Burrows, chair of the National Heart, Lung, and Blood Institute's Committee on Management of Asthma in the Elderly, "There are many practices, especially outside of fairly sophisticated pulmonary groups, in which anyone with chronic airflow obstruction from any cause is simply diagnosed as having COPD" (cited in Kyes, 1994).

Diagnostic testing for asthma should include pulmonary function studies, radiographic studies, blood draws for analysis of arterial blood gases (ABGs), and a complete blood count. In elderly patients, a differential diagnosis is also important. Other causes of dyspnea and wheezing such as congestive heart failure, pulmonary embolism, and gastroesophageal reflux disease must be ruled out. In interpreting these diagnostic tests, if the chest X-ray looks surprisingly normal for the degree of impairment experienced by the patient and no emphysematous changes are noted, an asthmatic component should be considered (Kyes, 1994). If the white blood count differential shows eosinophilia, the possibility of asthma is strong. Some studies have been conducted relating the immunoglobulin (IgE) level to asthma. Although the data are inconclusive, there seems to be some correlation between age-adjusted IgE serum levels and the presence of asthma (Hazzard et al., 1994). A pulmonary battery of ten skin tests is given in some situations. If the patients are highly **atopic** or have an inherited tendency to develop an allergy, then asthma is a more likely diagnosis (Kyes, 1994). Asthma should also be suspected as the cause of airflow obstruction if the symptoms are episodic (Hazzard et al., 1994).

The abnormalities in pulmonary function studies done on asthmatics may differ due to the episodic nature of the disease. Test results vary from patient to patient and with the same patient, depending on the severity of airflow obstruction on the day the test is conducted (Farzan, 1992). One useful diagnostic strategy for patients with episodic symptoms who test normal on spirometry is peak expiratory flow rate (PEFR) monitoring. Twice-daily PEFR measurements for several weeks may demonstrate variability in airflow obstruction. Marked improvement in postbronchodilator spirometry is indicative of asthma. Patients suspected of being asthmatic who fail to demonstrate reversibility after a bronchodilator may be given a 2-week treatment regimen of inhaled bronchodilators and oral corticosteroids. If there is a dramatic improvement in spirometry after the 2-week trial, the diagnosis of asthma is supported (Hazzard et al., 1994).

Unfortunately, there is nothing that excludes patients from having chronic bronchitis and/or emphysema as a result of smoking and also having asthma. These conditions often coexist in elderly asthmatics.

Arterial blood gas analysis helps identify asthmatics who require a hospital stay or aggressive therapy. During an asthmatic episode, ABGs are usually abnormal. The most common finding is mild to moderate hypoxemia with some degree of respiratory alkalosis. With more severe airway obstruction, hypoxemia may be more pronounced. When hypoxemia is accompanied by profound hypercapnia, a life-threatening situation exists, and patients need to be admitted to an acute care facility. A discussion of acute asthma can be found in Chapter 5.

Management. Management of asthma in older adults is based on the severity of the condition and on the presence or absence of comorbid conditions. Patients should be informed that asthma is a serious health problem.

All asthmatics over age 55 should be evaluated for coexisting circumstances that may cause complications (*JACI*, 1991). Heart disease, prostatism, cataracts, glaucoma, hypertension, and diabetes are all conditions that may be exacerbated by asthma drug therapy. Aspirin and nonsteroidal anti-inflammatory drugs (NSAIDS), used to alleviate arthritic pain, may precipitate bronchospasm. Chronic sinusitis seems to aggravate asthmatic symptoms in some patients (Hazzard et al., 1994). Environmental irritants such as industrial pollutants, smoke, wood or kerosene home heating, solvents found in closed offices, strong perfumes, and pets (especially cats and dogs) often exacerbate airflow obstruction.

Recognition of asthma triggers and knowing the early warning signs of an asthmatic episode are important in every age group. Management may simply consist of avoiding such triggers. With greater experience of what makes things better and worse for them, older persons may manage pretty well.

Pharmacological Intervention. Pharmacological intervention may include any or all of the following drug categories:

- Sympathomimetics
- Corticosteroids
- Anticholinergics
- Antiasthmatics
- Theophylline

These agents may be available in an oral form, in a liquid form for nebulization, or as metered-dose inhalers. Physicians prescribe various combinations of these drugs based on symptoms, patient tolerance, and comorbid conditions.

Successful treatment of asthma involves communication and cooperative efforts between the patient and the physician. Management of asthma must include education. Knowledge of environmental control, symptom recognition, and appropriate self-administration of drugs serve to achieve the ultimate goal of allowing older persons with asthma an opportunity to lead normal lives.

BRONCHIECTASIS

Bronchiectasis is another obstructive lung disease. It is characterized by irreversible dilation and destruction of the bronchial walls. Inflammatory processes or a localized infection can damage portions of the bronchial wall. The damaged ciliated epithelium is replaced by squamous epithelium (Witek and Schachter, 1994). Once the propulsive action of the cilia is lost in the involved area, defense mechanisms are altered. Patients with bronchiectasis have difficulty in mobilizing secretions. Eventually, bacteria colonize in the dilated, damaged bronchial wall. Secretions pool, and purulent sputum is present almost continuously.

In the past, bronchiectasis was often thought to be a consequence of severe viral respiratory infections such as measles and whooping cough. Today's older people did not enjoy the availability of vaccines against these common childhood diseases. Years ago, before the introduction of antibiotics, bronchial destruction also resulted from poorly resolved pneumonia (Witek and Schachter, 1994).

Although bronchiectasis is seen in all ages, its onset in the majority of patients was, and is, in childhood (Farzan, 1992). Currently, this disease is found primarily in patients who are predisposed to recurring pulmonary infections. This profile includes patients with abnormal immune systems, **agammaglobulinemia,** defective leukocyte function, or ciliary **dyskinesia,** also known as immotile cilia syndrome (Farzan, 1992). Patients in whom airway clearance is impaired—for example, by cystic fibrosis—account for nearly half of the bronchiectasis cases today. Tuberculosis and aspergillosis may also be associated with the development of bronchiectatic airways (Weinberger, 1986).

The course of this disease has changed. Improved control of recurrent infections with newer antibiotics has reduced the mortality rate and extended the life expectancy into the sixties and beyond. Unfortunately, as in other chronic lung diseases, progressive bronchiectasis is also accompanied by right ventricular heart failure, which is now the primary cause of disability and death.

Treatment.   Treatment of bronchiectasis is similar to that of other obstructive lung diseases. Two notable exceptions are the inclusion of chest physiotherapy (CPT) and antibiotics into the regimen. Postural drainage and CPT are particularly important to any patient with copious secretions. The frequency and duration of the drainage CPT depend on the severity of the disease, the amount of secretions, and the tolerance of the patient.

Antimicrobial drugs are regularly added to the protocol for bronchiectasis therapy as *Staphylococcus aureus* and pseudomonas are commonly isolated from the patient's sputum. In these patients, therapy should begin early in the course of an exacerbation, before systemic signs of infection are present. Some physicians prescribe continuous antibiotics in an attempt to keep the chronic infection under control. Continuous prophylaxis with antibiotics is, however, controversial (Dantzker et al., 1995).

Surgical resection has been used in some patients who present with a single localized area of damage, but with other treatments available, surgical resection of the diseased area is infrequent (Weinberger, 1986).

CYSTIC FIBROSIS

Cystic fibrosis is a hereditary, chronic lung disease. It has never been classified as a disease of the elderly because people with cystic fibrosis seldom live past the third decade of life. With recent discoveries, the possibility of gene therapy, new pharmacological agents, and heart-lung transplants, this may not be the case in the future.

REHABILITATION

As an adjunct to this section on chronic obstructive pulmonary diseases, any discussion of management strategies would not be complete without mentioning pulmonary rehabilitation. Many U.S. hospitals now have some component of rehabilitation incorporated into their services. Whether the rehabilitation program targets pulmonary or cardiac patients, or both, the results are generally positive.

Comprehensive pulmonary rehabilitation programs are designed to aid COPD and other respiratory disorder patients to adjust physically and psychologically to their disorder. Rehabilitation emphasizes lifestyle changes that enable patients to maximize their potential.

In the seventeenth century, Jeremy Taylor said, "To preserve a man alive in the midst of so many diseases and hostilities is as great a miracle as to create him." Preserving function in the presence of chronic impairment is a challenge to many respiratory care practitioners.

A complete review of rehabilitation techniques goes beyond the scope of the present chapter. There are many excellent books on rehabilitation that give comprehensive and in-depth information on the continuity of care after the acute phase of the disease has passed. Emphasis in this chapter is centered on the viability of rehabilitation programs for the elderly.

Unless there are existing exclusionary criteria, such as severe cardiac disease, life-limiting malignancy, or neurologic disability, advanced pulmonary disease should not prevent patients from some measure of participation. Too often, patients with chronic disorders become labeled by their disease and lose their identity. Rehabilitation programs often help individuals regain their sense of self. Once evaluated and assessed, elderly patients are very capable of participating in supervised exercise programs that have been tailored to meet their abilities. Educational sessions are incorporated in the program to help motivate individuals to maintain some degree of home exercise conditioning.

Although most rehabilitation programs are designed for noninstitutionalized patients, there is also a need for pulmonary rehabilitation in long-term care patients. For many years, the standard of care for pulmonary patients included inactivity and rest. Some long-term-care facilities have been successful in developing respiratory programs building on the concept of enablement. Enablement refers to care provisions that help the resident use and retain intact abilities and help to restore lost abilities. One program's agenda includes morning secretion clearance, therapeutic exercise, breathing control with exercise, and promotion of coping strategies. The alternate exercise-relaxation program has been beneficial in helping residents regain lost or absent abilities and function at a higher level (Taylor, Gleason, and Grady, 1995).

Age should not be an exclusionary factor for exercise, conditioning, or rehabilitation programs. The goal of encouraging individuals to maintain their highest functional level will result in a more balanced approach to health care for the elderly.

RESTRICTIVE LUNG DISEASE

Restrictive lung diseases are characterized by small, stiff lungs, a reduction in lung volumes, lung capacities, and lung compliance, and a gas exchange abnormality at the alveolar level.

Restrictive disorders may be subdivided into many categories based on etiology. They may present as acute or chronic processes. Some of the more common pulmonary restrictive diseases are:

- Pulmonary interstitial disease
- Pleural effusion
- Pneumothorax
- Cardiogenic pulmonary edema
- Noncardiogenic pulmonary edema, including acute respiratory distress syndrome (ARDS)
- Pneumonia
- Pulmonary embolism

INTERSTITIAL LUNG DISEASE

Pulmonary interstitial disorders, which are characterized by excessive tissue formed during the healing process of chronic or acute lung injury, comprise a large group of pulmonary disorders and are associated with pulmonary inflammatory changes (Des Jardins and Burton, 1995). When the inflammation is extensive, fibrosis, **granulomas,** or nodular inflammatory lesions and cavitation may result. Although there are no interstitial lung diseases that affect only the elderly, interstitial lung disease is common in later life (Hazzard et al., 1994). There are more than 140 different disease processes that are known to produce interstitial lung disorders (Des Jardins and Burton, 1995).

The most common disorders among the elderly are idiopathic pulmonary fibrosis, interstitial disease associated with collagen vascular disease, sarcoidosis, occupational lung diseases, hypersensitivity pneumonitis, and interstitial lung disease caused by drugs and irradiation (Hazzard et al., 1994).

Interstitial diseases, regardless of the cause, share two major pathologic components: an inflammatory process in the alveolar wall and a scarring or fibrotic process.

Diagnosis.   A chest X-ray is helpful in making a diagnosis. Characteristic films will show diffuse, bilateral densities, with increased linear and small nodular markings referred to as a reticulonodular pattern. Because up to 10 percent of patients with interstitial disease may have a normal X-ray, other diagnostic criteria are needed (Weinberger, 1986). Clinically these patients will present with fatigue, dyspnea on exertion, and often a chronic, nonproductive cough. Clubbing of the digits may be noted. Auscultation may reveal sharp crackling rales throughout the chest (Hazzard et al., 1994). Pulmonary function testing will show a reduction in volumes and a reduction in expiratory flows.

In establishing a diagnosis of interstitial disease, the patient needs a thorough history and physical examination in addition to a chest X-ray and PFTs. Occupational history may reveal as much as the physical exam and is especially important in aged patients. Exposure to some inorganic dusts, such as silica or asbestos, will not result in symptomatic lung disease until many years have passed. Benign pleural effusions, an early manifestation of an asbestos-related pulmonary disease, may not appear until 20 years after exposure (Dantzker, MacIntyre, and Bakow, 1995).

Arthritis.   Rheumatoid arthritis is a common interstitial lung disease associated with a collagen vascular disorder in the elderly. It is primarily an inflammatory joint disease, but it may involve the lungs (Des Jardins and Burton, 1995). It is usually mild, requiring no treatment (Hazzard et al., 1994).

Idiopathic Pulmonary Fibrosis.   Idiopathic pulmonary fibrosis, which implies unknown etiology, frequently occurs in older adults. Clinically most patients present with idiopathic pulmonary fibrosis between the ages of 40 and 70 (Weinberger, 1986). The prognosis for this disease is usually poor.

Pulmonary Sarcoidosis.   Pulmonary sarcoidosis is a multisystem, chronic, progressive granulomatous disease that may affect any part of the body. The lungs are frequently involved. Pulmonary sarcoidosis is usually diagnosed in younger people. It is, however, not unusual to detect sarcoidosis in older patients (Hazzard et al., 1994). Management is based on the severity of symptoms and the organs or tissues involved.

Drug-Induced Interstitial Lung Disease.   Drug-induced interstitial lung disease may be more common in the elderly population as a result of its etiology. Interstitial disorders may be identified as a result of a careful patient history. Radiation therapy for tumors of the breast, lung, or thorax may potentially cause this disease (Des Jardins and Burton, 1995). Many anticancer or antitumor agents used to treat malignancies may cause problems. Bleomycin and busulfan are the two cytotoxic agents associated with the highest incidence of interstitial lung disease (Hazzard et al., 1994).

Thoracoskeletal, Neurologic-Neuromuscular, and Abdominal Factors. In addition to pulmonary-restrictive disorders, chronic restriction of the lungs may also be caused by thoracoskeletal, neurologic-neuromuscular, and abdominal factors.

Any deformity of the thoracic cage that limits normal chest excursion is classified as a restrictive disorder. **Kyphosis,** a posterior curvature of the thoracic vertebrae, usually affects the spine at the top of the back. Kyphosis is often diagnosed in older individuals with degenerative osteoarthritis. Aging, osteoporosis, and steroid therapy have also been implicated as causative factors in the development of kyphosis. Not surprising is the fact that kyphosis may develop in patients with chronic obstructive pulmonary disease. **Kyphoscoliosis** is a combined deformity characterized by an anteroposterior curvature and lateral curvature of the spine. Any malalignment of the ribs and spine can interfere with proper ventilation.

Neurologic-Neuromuscular Restrictions. Neurologic-neuromuscular restrictions in elderly patients may be the result of paraplegia or quadriplegia, which of course knows no age barriers. **Hemiplegia,** paralysis of one side of the body, is most commonly associated in the elderly with stroke. A significant number of older patients contracted polio in their youth and are now dealing with postpolio syndrome. Muscular weakness appears to be a late complication of the infection. Whenever the diaphragm is affected there will be reduced lung volumes and a pattern of ventilation consistent with restrictive lung disease.

Abdominal-Restrictive Diseases. Abdominal-restrictive diseases are the result of limited diaphragmatic excursion, which is restricted by an overdistended or large abdomen. Obesity, for example, is a primary cause of such restriction. Pressure is applied to the abdominal muscles, which oppose the contraction of the diaphragm. **Ascites** is an abnormal accumulation of fluid within the peritoneal cavity. Ascites is usually a chronic condition that is hard to control. In the elderly it is associated with advanced congestive heart failure and liver failure. As in obesity, the pressure of the fluid in the peritoneal cavity ultimately slows the excursion of the diaphragm, resulting in limited lung expansion.

Therapy. Therapy and management in older patients diagnosed with restrictive interstitial lung disease is complicated by the high percentage of patients having other comorbid conditions. Treatment regimens vary with the specific diseases. In younger patients, antiinflammatory agents, usually corticosteroids, may alleviate some symptoms. In older patients the use of corticosteroids may aggravate other nonpulmonary-related illnesses. Sympathomimetics may be useful if there is any degree of smooth muscle contraction. Dyspnea in elderly patients with interstitial lung disease may be due to a diffusion defect or to capillary shunting. The hypoxemia caused by capillary shunting is relatively refractory to oxygen therapy. Dyspnea, on the other hand, may be due to comorbid conditions such as congestive heart failure in a patient with sarcoidosis. In this case, oxygen will make the patient more comfortable.

As a general statement, management is directed toward the inflammatory process of these pulmonary disorders or at the component that results in limited lung expansion.

CANCER

Cancer is the second-leading cause of death in the United States and the second-leading cause of death among the elderly. Increased longevity has led to an increased incidence of cancer. In comparing cancer sites relative to age, there are very few types that are not more prevalent as age increases (Table 4-1).

Cancer generally refers to abnormal tissue growth or uncontrolled growth and spread of cells. Human fibroblasts are genetically programmed to double about fifty times, which is called the *Hayflick limit,* after the scientist who first identified this phenomenon (Hayflick, 1974). He described the essential difference between normal tissues and cancers. Malignant growths (cancerous tumors or **neoplasms**) rapidly reproduce and continue to double and redouble past the fifty-doubling limit. Tumors literally take over their host.

TABLE 4-1   **Cancer Locations in Relation to Age**

Cancer Location	Age
Respiratory system	Among men, rates are highest at ages 45 to 64 compared with other cancers. Rates increase in both genders through age 75.
Digestive system	Rates are low under age 45. They increase rapidly thereafter for both sexes.
Female breast	Rates are highest of all cancers among women ages 25 to 54.
Male genital	Rates are high after age 65. They increase with age thereafter.
Female genital	Rates begin to increase after age 35. They increase more rapidly after age 55.
Urinary organs	Rates are low under age 55. Large increases occur later in life.
Leukemia	Rates are higher than other cancer rates in children but are still low. Rates increase dramatically after age 35.
Lymph and blood	This cancer is rare in children and young adults. Rates increase in middle years.

Source: *B. P. Hamann (1994).* Disease: Identification, prevention, and control. *St. Louis, MO: C. V. Mosby & Co., p. 324.*

Cellular regeneration is continually taking place as a normal process in the body. Cells reproduce regularly in order to replace damaged and worn-out tissue and to allow for growth and development of the body. For some reason cells often become altered. **Carcinogens,** loosely defined as cancer-causing substances, damage the genetic material of the cells. These altered cells relay incorrect or inappropriate genetic information, allowing new cells to proliferate in an abnormal, destructive manner. Neoplasms are the result of these growths.

Among the various types of cancer, lung cancer causes the most deaths: about 151,000 out of 538,000 annual cancer deaths, which represents about 28 percent of all cancer deaths and about 6.5 percent of total deaths (National Center for Health Statistics, 1996). There are about 170,000 new cases each year (Hamann, 1994). Of those who develop lung cancer, 83 percent are smokers. The long-term survival rate is slightly less than 10 percent.

Lung cancer used to be more prevalent in men than women. The increased frequency of smoking among women has, however, changed those statistics. By 1985, it was reported that there were more teenage females smoking than teenage males and that the death of women from lung cancer exceeded the number dying from breast cancer (May, 1991). Among those age 65 and older, 15.1 percent of males and 12.0 percent of females are current smokers, a significant decline over the years for males (from 36.4 percent in 1965) but a significant increase for females (from 9.6 percent in 1965; U.S. Bureau of the Census, 1994). The majority of lung cancer cases occur in patients over age 50 (Hazzard et al., 1994), with an increased rate in diagnosis between the ages of 65 and 75 (Hamann, 1994).

The causative factor for lung cancer has been identified and established to a greater degree than any other type of malignancy. Cigarette smoking is clearly responsible for the vast majority of cases, with environmental and occupational exposure identified as additional risks. The actual development of cancer as a result of smoking takes many years. Health care providers need to continue to be diligent in promoting smoking cessation.

TREATMENT

Treatment for lung cancer includes three forms of therapy: surgery, radiation, and chemotherapy. Early diagnosis will improve survival. Lung cancer, however, is often not detectable until it is fairly well advanced. The most common symptoms are a cough and **hemoptysis,** or spitting up blood.

Elderly patients seem to have a more localized disease when diagnosed. A greater proportion of older patients with cancer have squamous cell carcinoma (Figure 4-6), which is more resectable and thus more curable than other types (Hazzard et al., 1994). Operative and postoperative mortality rates in the aged tend to be higher. Small-cell carcinoma responds fairly well to radiation, but it is not as commonly diagnosed in the elderly (Figure 4-7). Although effective in many cases, chemotherapy may be risky among older adults due to age-related physiological changes and resultant changes in pharmacodynamics. Because of fear of toxicity, many physicians elect not to prescribe chemotherapy for older patients (Hazzard et al., 1994).

Respiratory care for patients diagnosed with lung cancer may involve modalities designed to mobilize secretions. Because of excessive mucus production and accumulation associated with lung cancer, aerosol and/or bronchodilator therapy may be beneficial. If atelectasis and alveolar consolidation are present, some form of hyperinflation therapy

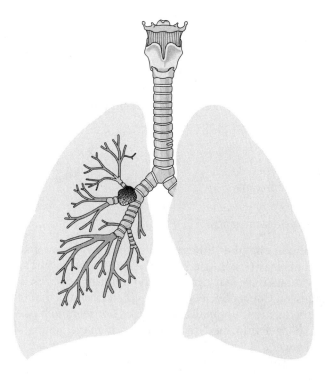

Figure 4-6 *Squamous cell carcinoma.* (Source: *From Barbara P. Hamann,* Disease: Identification, prevention, and control. *St. Louis: Mosby-Year Book, Inc., 1994. Reprinted by permission.)*

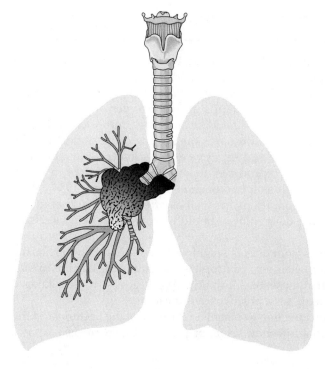

Figure 4-7 *Small-cell carcinoma.* (Source: *From Barbara P. Hamann,* Disease: Identification, Prevention, and Control. *St. Louis: Mosby-Year Book, Inc., 1994. Reprinted by permission.)*

may be useful. Oxygen therapy in some lung cancer patients may be therapeutic, but in others it may simply be palliative.

Cancers of the pancreas, stomach, colon, prostate, and breast all show age-specific increased rates (Hazzard et al., 1994). The risks and benefits of invasive versus noninvasive therapy must be carefully considered. Investigators continue in their quest to explain why older individuals are at greater risk for developing cancer. Some of the hypotheses are that older people:

- Have had a longer exposure to carcinogens
- Have more compromised immune systems
- Have an increased susceptibility to carcinogens
- Have a decreased ability to repair DNA
- Have an age-related loss of tumor suppressor genes

Diagnosis of cancer in older individuals may be difficult. Comorbid conditions may mask cancer symptoms. Cancer symptoms may be confused with the aging process and accepted as being normal. Elderly individuals may fear cancer to the point of not seeking medical help. For many years the American Cancer Society has provided free information on the warning signs of cancer. Since the incidence of malignancy does not seem to be decreasing, health care providers need to be well informed on prevention, management, and supportive care for older people with cancer.

TUBERCULOSIS

Once presumed to be nearly eradicated in the United States, tuberculosis has resurfaced. It kills about 1,300 people a year (National Center for Health Statistics, 1996).

Tuberculosis is caused by the aerobic bacillus *Mycobacterium tuberculosis*. The tuberculosis bacillus thrives in organs that have an abundant supply of oxygen, particularly the lungs. The bacillus, a rod-shaped bacterium, was first identified by Robert Koch in 1882. In the early part of the twentieth century, tuberculosis was the leading cause of death in the United States. Because of improved hygiene and selective elimination (people more susceptible to it had died off and thus did not reproduce), the incidence of death from tuberculosis by 1931 was only a quarter as high as it had been in 1880 (Herrman, 1934). With much-improved sanitation and living conditions, as well as effective chemotherapy, it would be a reasonable assumption that tuberculosis should be eradicated by now. However, this is not the case.

Transmission of tuberculosis comes from direct contact with an individual who has the disease. The primary infection occurs when aerosol droplets containing the bacillus are inhaled and reach the alveoli. The tuberculosis bacilli multiply very slowly. It often takes 4 to 10 weeks on laboratory culture media for a positive identification.

The extent of the posttransmission infection depends on the dose of the bacteria and the patient's general condition. The initial infection stage, or primary tuberculosis, may not manifest any symptoms at all. Upon initial exposure a mild or short illness may be seen in many patients. Symptoms may consist of a low-grade fever, loss of appetite, lethargy, and an occasional cough. The mildness of the symptoms in many infected individuals may go unnoticed and untreated. Without detection or treatment, the organisms remain in the body, where they slowly multiply. As part of the immune system's defense mechanism, macrophages engulf the bacteria but do not destroy them. Mycobacterium bacilli can remain dormant for many years and never develop into clinically active tuberculosis. In about 10 percent of the individuals to whom the disease is transmitted, the immune system is unable to limit the infection (Weinberger, 1986). This group of people will develop clinically apparent tuberculosis within 3 to 12 months.

Postsecondary tuberculosis, also known as reactivation tuberculosis, is caused by a reactivation of the dormant tuberculosis bacillus months or years after the initial infection (Des Jardins and Burton, 1995). In many instances, the reactivation occurs in people who are debilitated and have lower resistance to infection. At greatest risk for reactivation are older people, alcoholics, diabetics, immunosuppressed patients, nutritionally deficient individuals, and those with chronic debilitating disorders. Tuberculosis in patients with AIDS (acquired immune deficiency syndrome) is now at epidemic levels (Des Jardins and Burton, 1995). Tuberculosis in the elderly is on the rise, although the disease is both preventable and curable.

Contrary to a popular belief, once positive does not mean always positive in tuberculosis testing. In surveying large groups of elderly adults, it has been found that most were tuberculin negative, or nonimmune. Further investigation revealed that a majority of those same individuals had at one time or another been infected and had tested positive on the tuberculin test (Hazzard et al., 1994). With advanced age it appears that one change that takes place in the immune system is "loss of memory" of the T cells for the antigen. Thus, an individual who may have tested positive at age 40 could test negative at age 70. When older adults determined to be nonimmune (negative) convert to a positive test, further cultures are warranted. Tuberculosis must be considered a possibility in an older person with a pulmonary infection, especially if the individual has tested positive for it in the past (Hazzard et al., 1994).

Older people in long-term-care facilities may be at a higher risk for infection with *Mycobacterium tuberculosis.* Close living quarters and the chance that a diagnosis of tuberculosis in an elderly resident might be missed both contribute to the possibility of an outbreak of the disease. Studies have indicated that the typical symptoms of night sweats, fever, hemoptysis, and cough are more common in younger adults than older adults (Korzeniewska-Kosela et al., 1994). In a nursing home setting, if the symptoms of tuberculosis are not recognized or are mistakenly diagnosed as a pneumonic process, there is a strong possibility that additional cases will result.

Another consideration is the more common occurrence of miliary or disseminated tuberculosis in the elderly (Korzeniewska-Kosela et al., 1994), which may result from either reactivation tuberculosis or from a recent infection. Miliary or disseminated tuberculosis, as the name implies, is spread to other parts of the body by the blood. The infection is more systemic in disseminated tuberculosis, and the patient is usually quite ill. Miliary infections can involve bones, joints, meninges, lymph nodes, the liver, and can also cause tuberculosis pneumonia. This diagnosis is easily missed, not presenting the usual signs and symptoms of tuberculosis.

Spread of tuberculosis in long-term-care facilities not only puts residents at risk but endangers health care providers in these settings. Universal precautions should be emphasized.

PREVENTION AND TREATMENT

Prevention and treatment of tuberculosis can be accomplished with considerable efficacy. There is a vaccine available for tuberculosis, the BCG (bacille Calmette-Guérin) vaccine. Although some success has been achieved in providing partial immunity, the vaccine is not used routinely in the United States (Hamann, 1994). Even without the vaccine, tuberculosis is avoidable. Common-sense precautions include maintaining overall good health, avoiding deliberate exposure to tuberculosis, and participating in testing to detect the disease in its earliest stages.

Prevention of tuberculosis in long-term-care facilities mandates an effective surveillance program. Tuberculin status on admission should be established, and accurate records should be kept. An elderly patient who tests positive needs to have any respiratory infection investigated by doing sputum cultures. In the event that the sputum does grow *Mycobacterium tuberculosis,* treatment should be initiated.

Multidrug regimens are the most effective means of treating tuberculosis. In order to prevent the growth of drug-resistant strains of tuberculosis, two or even three antituberculous agents may be prescribed. The suggested regimen in newly diagnosed older patients is isoniazid and rifampin daily for 9 months (Hazzard et al., 1994). Ethambutol is also very effective, but adding a third drug may precipitate a toxic reaction in the elderly. When confronted with cases of confusion of recent onset in older adults, experienced geriatricians always consider the possibility of a drug reaction.

Outpatient therapy in noninstitutionalized older people involves the same drugs. Because definitive diagnosis depends on bacteriological confirmation, the diagnosis must often be made on suspicion, and treatment must be started before a positive diagnosis is obtained (Davies, 1994).

The patient should be told that the proper dosage of the drug must be taken regularly for the duration of therapy in order to be effective. Treatment failures occur as a result of failure to comply with the drug regimen, failure of the drug, or failure of the physician to prescribe the correct medication in adequate amounts (Hazzard et al., 1994).

Surveillance during the course of therapy will indicate the effectiveness of the antitubercular agents and monitor for adverse reactions. Sputum cultures should be done periodically until the acid-fast bacilli culture is negative. Adverse drug reactions may manifest as nausea, vomiting, anorexia, or jaundice. If toxicity is suspected, the serum glutamic oxaloacetic transaminase (SGOT) level, now known as asparate aminotransferase (AST), should be measured. If elevated, hepatic toxicity is likely. In most cases, reduction in drug dosages will return AST to normal. About 90 percent of elderly patients tolerate isoniazid without difficulty (Hazzard et al., 1994). Prophylactic chemotherapy is also used under certain circumstances. Isoniazid preventive therapy may be prescribed to some at-risk patients as a precautionary measure.

SUMMARY

There are numerous chronic diseases in the elderly that could be discussed in this chapter—diseases that do not directly affect the cardiopulmonary system but might be of significance to the respiratory care practitioner. Diabetes, Parkinson's disease, and Alzheimer's disease, as well as many other chronic illnesses, may directly or indirectly affect pulmonary function. The possibility of comorbid conditions in older people must always be considered, as must the course of chronic conditions. One may lead to another. A person with arthritis, for example, may develop pneumonia. A person institutionalized with a broken hip may become infected with tuberculosis in the nursing home. It would be impossible to cover all of the various conditions or combinations of conditions that might impact on pulmonary care in some way.

As people grow older they do not become more alike; they demonstrate more differences (see Chapter 1). Older people with chronic diseases are not all alike. For one thing, they are not all sick or disabled. They may not exhibit detectable symptoms, or the symptoms they have may not be all that similar to those of younger people with the same conditions. Pneumonia, for example, may present as an entirely different kind of disease in the elderly. Similarly, older people do not always respond in the same manner to therapy.

Some older people may consider signs and symptoms of chronic illness to simply be a part of the aging process. A certain number of aches and pains and disabilities have come to be accepted by many individuals as part of old age. Often, symptoms that would demand immediate attention in a younger person may be ignored later in life. The complications of disease that are overlooked frequently have unfortunate outcomes. Infection, for example, can be a cause of confusion in later life. Confusional states among the aged are assumed to be dementia and too often are dismissed as irreversible. One psychiatrist has said that over two-thirds of the patients he saw who were admitted for delirium in fact had an undiagnosed infection of one kind or another (Eisdorfer, 1972).

A discussion in Chapter 8 addresses the fact that some older people are ambivalent as to whether or not they wish life to continue. These individuals may present with an entirely different pattern of seeking—or avoiding—health care regimens and compliance.

Caring for elderly patients involves direct communication. It must be taken into consideration that many older adults have some degree of sensory impairment. Older patients are occasionally confused by their new environment. Kindness and consideration are due to all patients, but with older adults a few modifications will usually improve the efficacy of their treatment. Caregiving tips for elderly patients include the following:

1. Always identify yourself in a calm and unhurried manner.
2. Direct eye contact and a lower tone of voice will increase the likelihood that the patient understands instructions.
3. Be patient.
4. When assessing patients, accept the fact that if the pulse and respiratory rate are irregular, which they often are, they should be counted for a full minute to assure accuracy.
5. If the patient is frightened by having a nebulizer strapped to his or her face, do *not* do it. Holding the mask close to the patient's nose and mouth will accomplish the same goal.

6. If the patient cannot easily actuate his or her metered-dose inhaler, seek ways to modify the procedure. Prior to dismissal, have the patient give you a return demonstration to verify his or her ability to take the prescribed medication.
7. Be culturally sensitive. If language is a barrier, find an interpreter—ideally, a family member. Fear and confusion will only add to the patient's breathing problems.
8. Never underestimate the power of touch. Letting patients hold your hand during the treatment may have therapeutic benefits.
9. Always be diligent about handwashing.

The changing distribution of the American population by age has placed greater demands on the health care system. The field of geriatric medicine and geriatric patient care ranges anywhere from common sense to high tech. Biomedical researchers and health promotion specialists are continually seeking ways to eliminate or postpone the chronic diseases associated with the aging process. Health care providers must seek out educational opportunities to learn about care of the aged. Former Surgeon General of the United States C. Everett Koop once said, "Elderly care, when the practitioner is motivated and well versed in contemporary geriatric practice, can help make aging a living process, not a dying one" (Olson and Young, 1992).

Review Questions

1. Describe examples of how diet and stress contribute to the incidence of coronary artery disease.
2. Your neighbor's 78-year-old father has just been diagnosed as having COPD. She asks you what to expect. How will you answer her?
3. Why do you think some elderly patients delay seeking a diagnosis or treatment for cancer?
4. What are the warning signs of an impending stroke?
5. Should worldwide tuberculosis screening be instituted? Should screening be reinstated in the United States?

References

American Lung Association (1993). *Asthma—At my age?* Washington, DC: National Council on the Aging.

Barrow, G. M. (1989). *Aging, the individual, and society.* St. Paul, MN: West.

Bloom, G. M., and Schlom, E. A. (1993). *Drug prescribing for the elderly.* New York: Raven Press.

Coyle, K. A., Smith, R. B., Salam, A. A., Dodson, T. F., et al. (1994). Carotid endarterectomy in the octogenarian. *Annals of Vascular Surgery, 8,* 417–420.

Dantzker, D. R., MacIntyre, N. R., and Bakow, E. D. (1995). *Comprehensive respiratory care.* Philadelphia: W. B. Saunders.

Davies, P. D. (1994). Tuberculosis in the elderly. *Journal of Antimicrobial Chemotherapy, 34* (supplement A), 93–100.

Des Jardins, T., and Burton, G. G. (1995). *Clinical manifestations and assessment of respiratory disease.* St. Louis: Mosby.

Eisdorfer, C. (1972). The impact of scientific advances on independent living. In J. Thorson (Ed.), *Action for older Americans toward independent living.* Athens: University of Georgia Center for Continuing Education, pp. 44–51.

Farzan, S. (1992). *A concise handbook of respiratory diseases,* 3rd ed. Norwalk, CT: Appleton & Lange.

Freiberg, K. L. (1992). *Human development: A life-span approach.* Boston: Jones and Bartlett.

Giordano, M. (1993, Nov.). Assessing the needs of geriatric patients at home. *AARC Times, 17* (11), 52–54.

Haddad, A. M. (1987). *High tech home care.* Rockville, MD: Aspen.

Hamann, B. P. (1994). *Disease: Identification, prevention, and control.* St. Louis: Mosby.

Hawkins, D. W., Hall, W. D., and Douglas, M. B. (1994). A multicenter analysis of the use of enalapril and lisinopril in elderly hypertensive patients. *Journal of the American Geriatrics Society, 42,* 1273–1276.

Hayflick, L. (1974). The strategy of senescence. *The Gerontologist, 14,* 37–45.

Hazzard, W. R., Bierman, E. L., Blass, J. P., Ettiger, W. H., and Halter, J. B. (Eds.) (1994). *Principles of geriatric medicine and gerontology.* New York: McGraw-Hill.

Herrman, C. (1934). Selective elimination as a factor in increasing the immunity of populations. A decade of progress in eugenics. *Scientific papers of the Third International Congress of Eugenics.* Baltimore: Williams & Wilkins.

Hogstel, M. O. (1994). *Nursing care of the older adult,* 3rd ed. Albany, NY: Delmar.

Journal of Allergy and Clinical Immunology (1991, Supplement). Guidelines for the diagnosis and management of asthma: National Heart, Lung, and Blood Institute National Asthma Education Program Expert Panel Report. St. Louis: Mosby Year Book.

Kacmarek, R. M., Mack, C. W., and Dimas, S. (1990). *The essentials of respiratory care,* 3rd ed. St. Louis: Mosby Year Book.

Korzeniewska-Kosela, M., Krysl, J., Muller, N., Black, W., et al. (1994). Tuberculosis in young adults and the elderly—A prospective comparison study. *Chest, 106,* 28–32.

Kyes, K. (1994). Geriatric asthma: A conversation with Benjamin Burrows, MD. *RT—The Journal for Respiratory Care Practitioners, 7* (3), 31–35.

Levitzky, M. G., Cairo, J. M., and Hall, S. M. (1990). *Introduction to respiratory care.* Philadelphia: W. B. Saunders.

Lucas, J., Golish, J. A., Sleeper, G., and O'Ryan, J. A. (1988). *Home respiratory care.* Norwalk, CT: Appleton & Lange.

Marieb, E. N. (1992). *Human anatomy and physiology,* 2nd ed. Redwood City, CA: Benjamin/Cummings.

Martin, D. E. (1988). *Respiratory anatomy and physiology.* St. Louis: C. V. Mosby.

May, D. F. (1991). *Rehabilitation and continuity of care in respiratory disease.* St. Louis: Mosby Year Book.

National Center for Health Statistics (1996, October 4). *Monthly Vital Statistics Report, 45* (3), Supplement 2, p. 29.

Needham, J. F. (1993). *Gerontological nursing: A restorative approach.* Albany, NY: Delmar.

O'Donnell, D. E., Webb, K. A., and McGuire, M. A. (1993). Older patients with COPD: Benefits of exercise training. *Geriatrics, 48,* 59–66.

O'Donohue, W. J. (1988). The future of home oxygen therapy. *Respiratory Care, 33,* 1125–1130.

O'Donohue, W. J., and Plummer, A. L. (1995). Magnitude of usage and cost of home oxygen therapy in the United States. *Chest, 107,* 301–302.

Olson, E. A., and Young, R. F. (1992). Continuing education in geriatrics: An imperative for elderly care. *The Journal of Continuing Education in the Health Professions, 12,* 25–32.

Ornish, D. (1993). *Eat more, weigh less.* New York: HarperCollins.

Reiss, B. S., and Evans, M. E. (1993). *Pharmacological aspects of nursing care* (4th ed.). Albany, NY: Delmar.

Stedman, S. (1994). *Concise medical dictionary.* Baltimore: Williams & Wilkins.

Taylor, J. S., Gleason, J., and Grady, L. (1995). An innovative approach to respiratory management for long-term-care patients. *The Gerontologist, 35,* 267–270.

Thorson, J. A. (1995). *Aging in a changing society.* Belmont, CA: Wadsworth.

Tierney, L. M., McPhee, S. J., and Papadakis, M. A. (1995). *Current medical diagnosis and treatment.* Norwalk, CT: Appleton & Lange.

U.S. Bureau of the Census (1994). *Statistical Abstract of the United States, 1994* (114th edition). Washington, D.C., 1994.

Walsh, K. (1994). Guidelines for the prevention and control of tuberculosis in the elderly. *Nurse Practitioner, 19* (11), 79–84.

Weinberger, S. E. (1986). *Principles of pulmonary medicine.* Philadelphia: W. B. Saunders.

Witek, T. J., and Schachter, N. E. (1994). *Pharmacology and therapeutics in respiratory care.* Philadelphia: W. B. Saunders.

CHAPTER FIVE

PHARMACOLOGY

—————— KEY TERMS ——————

beta-agonist
bioavailability
biotransformation
cumulation
cytosol

drug duplication
first-pass effect
hypoxemia
hypoxia

pharmacodynamics
pharmacokinetics
polypharmacy
protein-bound

—————— LEARNING OBJECTIVES ——————

After completing this chapter, the reader should be able to:

1. Define the stages of pharmacokinetics and discuss how and why age-related changes in the elderly alter these processes.
2. Define pharmacodynamics and discuss changes in drug action that relate to aging.
3. Describe the more common adverse drug reactions that affect the elderly.
4. Explain why polypharmacy is more prevalent in the older population.

INTRODUCTION

Geriatric pharmacology is a subject that all health care providers, including respiratory care practitioners, need in their education and training. The prevalence of drug use among older people is significant. Although only 13 percent of the U.S. population is age 65 or older, they account for over 30 percent of the total annual national expenditure for prescription drugs (Gleason, 1996). It has been projected that by the year 2030 the older population will account for over 40 percent of drug expenditures nationally (Chalker and Celli, 1993). It has also been estimated that 70 percent of older adults regularly use over-the-counter (OTC) medications. In addition, 20 to 25 percent of the hospitalizations of patients over age of 65 are the result of adverse drug reactions (Reiss and Evans, 1993). Although research is underway and the knowledge base of geriatric pharmacology is expanding, there is still much to be learned about medication usage among older people.

SUCCESSFUL DRUG THERAPY

When a patient is seen by his or her physician and a diagnosis is made, the most likely outcome will be a prescription for one or more medications. Successful drug therapy in later life exemplifies the importance of an interdisciplinary team being vigilant in their respective roles. Physicians who prescribe and patients who consume drugs are dependent on the health care team members. Pharmacists, nurses, therapists, and other caregivers involved in any medication transaction must assure that the drugs are delivered in a timely and accurate fashion. The goal is to ensure that maximum benefits are derived from drug therapy. When that goal is achieved, the potential exists for an enhanced quality of life and quality of care for the patient.

Geriatric pharmacotherapy requires knowledge of various aspects of the aging process. Advanced age increases vulnerability to disease and alters responses to pharmacologic agents. Since all medications are capable of causing adverse effects, the potential benefits must outweigh the potential risks. The primary goal of drug therapy with older adults is to improve the quality of life. A drug is any substance, other than food, used in the prevention, diagnosis, alleviation, treatment, or cure of disease (McDonough, 1993). Drugs fall into two categories: therapeutic drugs used in the treatment of disease, and palliative drugs that alleviate symptoms. Planning and implementing safe drug therapy, either for therapeutic or palliative purposes, begins with an understanding of **pharmacokinetics** and **pharmacodynamics.** The overall effect of the drug on the body is closely related to the action of the body on the drug.

PHARMACOKINETICS

Pharmacokinetics is the way in which a drug is handled within the body. The four phases of pharmacokinetics are absorption into the bloodstream, distribution throughout the body, metabolism or **biotransformation,** and excretion or elimination. Physiological changes in the body due to the aging process affect pharmacokinetics. The end result may be a higher or lower concentration of the drug at the site of action.

ABSORPTION

In order for a drug to cause a reaction, it must reach a receptor or target site. In order to reach a target site, the drug must first cross cell membranes, such as in the epithelial lining of the gastric mucosa or pulmonary mucosa. Cell membranes are composed of a double lipid layer of molecules sandwiched between two polypeptide layers. Receptors are proteins that serve as recognition sites for various stimuli. Most receptors are found in the cell's double lipid membrane. Cell membranes are also perforated by small pores, which allow for filtration of smaller molecules (Rau, 1994). Transport of substances across the cell membrane is most commonly achieved by passive diffusion, which relies on a concentration gradient. Lipid solubility, ionization, and molecule size are all factors that influence, and perhaps even prevent, drug diffusion across cell membranes. Once across the membrane, the drug reaches the bloodstream—unless through intravenous (IV) access the drug has already been injected directly into the bloodstream. In order to achieve their desired effect, many drugs need to cross an additional membrane, the blood–brain barrier. The blood–brain barrier is not readily permeable to electrolytes or ions.

Parkinson's disease is one of the major dementing illnesses in later life, third in frequency after Alzheimer's disease and multi-infarct dementia. Parkinson's is caused by a lack of dopamine-containing neurons in the central nervous system (CNS). A current approach to treating Parkinsonism is to increase the level of dopamine in the CNS. However, dopamine does not pass through the blood–brain barrier. Treatment may be accomplished by administering the drug levodopa (L-dopa), which will cross the blood–brain barrier. It is then converted to dopamine by decarboxylation. A newer drug that combines carbidopa with L-dopa (Sinemet) is also being used to effectively cross the blood–brain barrier and produce dopamine in the CNS.

Route of Administration.   The route of drug administration plays a role in absorption, particularly among the elderly.

Oral Administration.   There are several age-related changes in the gastrointestinal (GI) tract. Healthy older adults have been found to have hypochlorohydria, an increased gastric pH as a result of decreased gastric acid secretions. Older people also have a decreased splanchnic blood flow, decreased gastric emptying, and a decreased **first-pass effect,** leading to increased drug availability in the systemic system (Lamy, 1990). The first-pass effect relates to drugs administered orally. Drugs absorbed through the gastric mucosa are immediately delivered by the portal circulation to the liver. Enzymes in the liver metabolize the drugs, sometimes slowly, sometimes very rapidly. Rapid metabolism decreases the **bioavailability,** or portion of the drug that reaches the systemic circulation. Slow metabolism would then result in increased bioavailability. The use of stimulant laxatives, however—a common practice among many older adults—accelerates the movement of drugs through the GI tract, thus shortening the absorption phase. The decreased gastric pH may delay the breakdown and dissolution of tablets given orally. The decrease in gastric motility will prolong the absorption phase of the drug. All of these potential factors must be taken into consideration with the oral administration of drugs.

Intramuscular Absorption.   Intramuscular (IM) absorption of medications has not been extensively studied in the aged (Beizer, 1994). Based on what is known about age-related physiological changes, however, some predictions on absorption can be made:

1. Patients with peripheral vascular disease have a reduced blood flow.
2. There is an increased amount of connective tissue in aging muscle.
3. Elderly people have a reduction in lean muscle mass.
4. Lean muscle mass reduction in the elderly is compensated for by an increase in the amount of body fat.

These combined factors may impair the absorption of IM injections and may impair the permeability of tissue to injected drugs, decreasing systemic dissipation. Reduction of muscle mass may also make IM injections difficult to administer and painful for the patient.

Transdermal Absorption. Age-related changes in the skin may present obstacles to transdermal absorption of medications. These changes include:

1. Loss of water
2. A decreased number of cells in the dermis
3. A slight calcification of the elastic fibers in the dermis
4. A general overall skin thinning
5. A generalized reduction in perfusion to the skin

Efficacy of transdermal products in the elderly has not undergone extensive study and is open to further research.

Aerosolization. Aerosolized medications widely used in respiratory care are well absorbed by the lung mucosa if the airway is patent (Howder, 1992; Figure 5-1). Aging, however, causes changes in the structure and function of the respiratory system. These changes include a loss of alveolar elastic recoil; alterations in the chest wall structure, causing decreased compliance; decreased respiratory muscle strength; and loss of alveolar surface area and capillary blood volume (Levitzky, 1991). Age-related changes, coupled with chronic disease states, may result in a large ventilation-perfusion abnormality that will affect the absorption of a drug through the alveolar-capillary membrane. Although a quantity of the drug may be lost to nonperfused, nonventilated areas, aerosolization is still an effective means of drug administration (Howder, 1992).

DISTRIBUTION

Drug distribution in the aged may vary considerably from that in younger patients. Age-related changes affecting drug distribution include reduction of total body water, atrophy of muscle tissue with a resultant increase in the percentage of fatty tissue, and a generalized decrease in the protein-binding capability of drugs (Reiss and Evans, 1993). Loss of water may affect the distribution of water-soluble drugs such as aminoglycosides (gentamicin, streptomycin, tobramycin), lithium, and cimetidine, causing higher serum concentrations in the older patient. The use of diuretics further exacerbates the problem. An increase in the percent of body fat can alter the distribution of fat-soluble drugs. Some hypnotic agents and sedatives, barbiturates, phenothiazines, benzodiazepines, and phenitoin are fat soluble, leading to the potential storage of the drug in fatty deposits and resulting in an increased half-life (Hogstel, 1994).

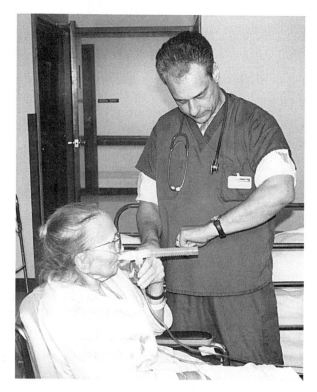

Figure 5-1 *Aerosolization is an effective means of drug administration.*

Some pharmaceutical agents are highly **protein bound**—that is, bound in plasma to the protein albumin and not biologically active. Use of drugs such as warfarin, furosemide, and diazepam may potentially be cause for concern. Serum albumin concentrations are normally reduced as a consequence of aging (Table 5-1). When serum albumin is reduced, the protein binding sites are likewise reduced, thus allowing for free biologically active drugs in circulation. An increased amount of warfarin in circulation could lead to hemorrhage, especially in older people. As Miller (1994) explains, "Recent studies conclude that warfarin is beneficial for the prevention of stroke in patients with atrial fibrillation—but caution is based on indications that the anticoagulant response is exaggerated in older patients—on the basis of age itself" (pp. 167–168).

METABOLISM

The biotransformation of drugs is a process by which drugs that enter the body are altered, inactivated, and prepared for elimination (Bills and Soderberg, 1994). This biotransformation depends on the activity of hepatic enzymes, hepatic blood flow, and the number of functioning liver cells, all of which are naturally reduced in older patients. Biotransformation, or metabolism, occurs through enzymatic reactions, primarily in the liver, but may occur in other organs as well, such as the lungs, kidneys, and intestines, or in the bloodstream.

TABLE 5-1 **Factors Affecting Pharmacokinetics in Older Patients**

	Normal Aging	**Disease States**
Absorption	No change affecting drug	Malabsorption
		Pancreatitis
	↑ gastric pH	Gastric surgery
	↓ gastrointestinal motility	
	↓ gastrointestinal blood flow	
Distribution	↓ total body water	Congestive heart failure
	↓ lean body mass	
	↓ serum albumin	Hepatic or renal insufficiency
	↑ body fat	
Hepatic metabolism	↓ liver size	Congestive heart failure
	↓ liver blood flow	
	↓ enzyme activity	Thyroid disease
		Cancer
Renal clearance	↓ renal blood flow	Volume depletion
	↓ glomerular filtration	Chronic renal insufficiency
	↓ tubular secretion	

Source: *M. O. Hogstel (1994).* Nursing care of the older adult. *Albany, NY: Delmar.*

One drug commonly prescribed for elderly patients with chronic obstructive pulmonary disease (COPD) is theophylline. Eighty-five to ninety percent of theophylline is metabolized in the liver (Spratto and Woods, 1993). Potential adverse side effects are of particular concern in older patients. Multifocal atrial tachycardia occurs with a higher incidence in the elderly, and it may be an early sign of theophylline toxicity (Bloom and Schlom, 1993). Tachycardia and arrhythmias associated with theophylline are strongly related to the drug level. Cigarette smoking has been shown to induce hepatic enzyme activity (Hogstel, 1994). Older smokers, therefore, would metabolize theophylline more rapidly, resulting in lower serum levels of the drug. Dietary changes, antacids, and tube feedings may result in erratic absorption of oral theophylline. Conditions such as viral infections, heart failure, cor pulmonale, and hypoxia all increase theophylline levels and predispose the patient to toxicity (Bloom and Schlom, 1993). Because hepatic metabolism is highly variable from individual to individual, particularly in elderly patients with diminished hepatic enzymes, dosage alteration is suggested (Hogstel, 1994). It is recommended that the dosage of theophylline in older adults be adjusted to maintain the serum level at the lower end of the usual therapeutic range, around 12 mg/ml (Bloom and Schlom, 1993).

RENAL EXCRETION

The last phase of pharmacokinetics is elimination of the drug from the body, either in its unaltered form or as a metabolite. The kidneys serve as the most important organs in drug elimination. Renal excretion is considered the most important pharmacokinetic change in older people (Beizer, 1994). With aging, there is a gradual decline in renal function, believed to be due to reduced blood flow to the kidneys or the loss of intact nephrons (Reiss and Evans, 1993). Between the fourth and eighth decade of life, renal mass decreases an average of 20 percent, and renal blood flow decreases by 10 ml/min per decade after age 30 (Bennett, 1990). Reduced renal blood flow, reduced glomerular filtration, and reduced tubular secretions are all part of the normal aging process. Any of these conditions may seriously impair the body's ability for drug clearance, which could lead to **cumulation,** a condition in which the rate of drug elimination is slower than the rate of drug administration. In patients with renal failure or impaired kidney function, cumulation could cause drug toxicity.

The creatinine clearance (CrCl), a measure of kidney function, also declines in a linear fashion with the aging process beginning in the forties (Bennett, 1990). Measuring CrCl via a 24-hour urine collection is the most accurate way of assessing renal function in older people, but obviously it is not the easiest or most practical method. Cockcroft and Gault (1976) developed equations to estimate CrCl by factoring in the patient's age, lean body weight (LBW), serum creatinine (SCr) level, and gender:

$$\text{CrCl (ml/min) male} = \frac{(140 - \text{age}) \ (\text{LBW in kg})}{72 \times \text{SCr}}$$

$$\text{CrCl (ml/min) female} = \text{CrCl male} \times 0.85$$

These equations have been useful in calculating dosages for drugs that are eliminated by glomerular filtration. Identification of patients with reduced CrCl should precipitate an appropriate modification in drug dosage—either a reduced dose or a longer interval between dosages (Beizer, 1994). Keep in mind, though, that even with the use of calculations and an estimated CrCl to alter drug dosages, it is still essential to monitor elderly patients closely for the development of drug toxicity related to the accumulation of drugs in the body.

PHARMACODYNAMICS

Pharmacodynamics, unlike pharmacokinetics, does not lend itself to any form of direct measurement—as in renal function assessment by measurement of serum creatinine. Pharmacodynamics refers to the activity of a drug when it interacts with a target site, receptor, or end organ. Receptors for drugs that act on the respiratory system have been subclassified as alpha and beta. The action of acetylcholine on receptors has also been identified as either muscarinic or nicotinic. An important aspect of respiratory care focuses on drugs that are active at more than one receptor type (Witek and Schachter, 1994).

SYMPATHOMIMETICS

In respiratory care, one of the primary modes of drug administration is aerosolization, either by small-volume nebulizers or metered-dose inhalers. The drugs most commonly aerosolized are **beta-agonists.** The receptors responsive to beta-agonists are molecular in size and are found, among other places, in the bronchial smooth muscles. The reaction of a beta-agonist on a beta-receptor results in bronchodilation. Although the data on beta-receptor responsiveness in the aged population are conflicting, most studies demonstrate that older people have a decreased beta-receptor sensitivity. Aging tends to decrease hormone responsiveness in several receptor systems.

Research done by Feldman and his colleagues (1984) at the University of Iowa hospitals and clinics has yielded some interesting data. They found that the aged seem to have an overall reduced beta-adrenergic sensitivity and reduced sensitivity to beta-agonists, without any concomitant reduction in receptor density or numbers of receptors. The reduction in beta-responsiveness was demonstrated by a decreased cardiac response to a beta-agonist, isoproterenol, and a decreased response to a beta-antagonist, propranalol. Receptor numbers remained stable, suggesting an alteration in the receptor-adenyl cyclase system. Further research linking the catecholamine level in adults ages 21 to 74 with beta-receptor responsiveness demonstrated that with advancing age there was an increase in the plasma norepinephrine level and a reciprocal reduction in beta-receptor affinity for agonists. Despite inconclusive evidence as to the status of beta-receptors in the elderly, pre- and postbronchodilator studies continue to demonstrate improvement in older adults who use sympathomimetics.

Current recommended dosages for beta-agonists in older patients remain the same as dosages for younger adults. Few studies have evaluated pharmacodynamic alterations of medications in the aged (Bloom and Schlom, 1993).

ANTICHOLINERGICS

Postmaturational changes in responsiveness have also been demonstrated in the muscarinic-acetylcholine receptor system. It is mainly the exposure to agonists, however, that causes these receptors to become selectively refractory to further stimulation (Scarpace, 1988). Muscarinic antagonists or anticholinergics have been used as bronchodilators since the seventeenth century. It is now well established that inhaled anticholinergic therapy is effective in treating chronic obstructive pulmonary disease (Chalker and Celli, 1993). There are two main subclasses of anticholinergics: atropine, a tertiary ammonia compound; and ipratropium bromide, a quaternary ammonia compound.

Tertiary ammonia compounds are absorbed readily across the blood–brain barrier and cause systemic side effects. The quaternary compounds are poorly absorbed and do not cross the blood–brain barrier, thus causing few systemic side effects. The muscarinic antagonist, ipratropium bromide, is widely used in respiratory therapy, especially now that ipratropium (Atrovent) is available in solution for nebulization. Bronchodilation using these agents is achieved by blocking the action of the parasympathetic system, which effectively decreases the level of cyclic guanosine monophosphate (GMP), a nucleotide that causes bronchoconstriction. The distinction between atropine and ipratropium bromide is important, especially in elderly patients. They seem to have an elevated susceptibility to the side effects of anticholinergics (Beizer, 1994).

Dry eyes and a dry mouth are common side effects of anticholinergics and may be more pronounced and more bothersome in the aged. Patients already suffering from constipation or urine retention may find that the use of an anticholinergic, atropine in particular, may make their symptoms worse.

GLUCOCORTICOIDS

Nearly all drugs produce their effect by reaching a target receptor. Most receptors are located in the double lipid layered cell membrane. The receptors for corticosteroids, on the other hand, are located in the cell **cytosol,** the liquid medium of the cytoplasm. Hormones or drugs specific for these receptors must thus penetrate the cell in order to effect binding (Witek and Schachter, 1994). These receptors are found in virtually all cells. Glucocorticoids influence a variety of body mechanisms. Cortisol, a naturally produced hormone from the adrenal cortex, is the most important endogenous glucocorticoid. It affects practically every organ system. The anti-inflammatory properties of glucocorticoids have made them useful in treating respiratory problems. Asthma, which researchers now suggest is a persistent bronchitis in which inflammation of the mucous membranes is present, responds well to corticosteroid therapy (Witek and Schachter, 1994). Because receptors for corticosteroids are so widespread throughout the body, adverse systemic side effects with complications are common. The introduction of inhaled steroids delivered via metered-dose inhalers reduced, but did not totally eliminate, untoward side effects.

Bloom and Schlom (1993) have compiled information concerning the treatment of elderly respiratory patients with systemic steroids. Possible adverse effects include the potential for serious infection in older patients, for example, reactivation of tuberculosis or cutaneous zoster. Patients should be screened for latent tuberculosis and receive prophylaxis when indicated. Potential side effects of prolonged systemic corticosteroids include:

- Myopathy
- Moon face
- Weight gain
- Adrenal suppression
- Osteoporosis
- Hypokalemia
- Hypertension
- Poor wound healing
- Peptic ulcer disease
- Confusion
- Posterior cataracts
- Psychosis
- Increased intraocular pressure

There are also some potential drug interactions with the use of steroids:

- Rifampin and anticonvulsants decrease the pharmacologic effects of steroids.
- Exogenous estrogen and cimetidine can enhance the effects of steroids.

- Concomitant use of nonsteroidal anti-inflammatory drugs (NSAIDS) with corticosteroids can precipitate increased gastrointestinal toxicity.
- Diuretics and steroids combined can increase the severity of hypokalemia.

Systemic steroids should be tapered to avoid withdrawal symptoms. Withdrawal symptoms may be nonspecific complaints including vague aches and pains, lethargy, and anorexia, all of which could easily be overlooked in older patients.

Aerosolized Steroids. Aerosolized steroids have the potential to eliminate or significantly reduce usage of systemic steroids and concomitant side effects. Their disadvantages include adverse effects such as cough, sore throat, and bronchospasm. The bronchospasm can be lessened by pretreatment with a sympathomimetic bronchodilator, or by switching to another inhaled steroid. Oral candidiasis (thrush) can be averted by using a spacer and/or rinsing out the mouth after inhaling the steroid.

The main potential problem with the use of metered-dose inhalers in the elderly—the only delivery mode of inhaled steroids—is the skill and coordination required for optimal benefit (Figure 5-2). The addition of spacers and specially designed adapters for patients with arthritis are helpful. Adverse effects of steroid use in the elderly may not be related to pharmacodynamic changes associated with the receptors, but rather with the interaction of steroids and other pharmaceutical agents used to treat disease processes common to older patients.

When administering medications to elderly patients, the pharmacokinetic and pharmacodynamic alterations must be kept in mind. When consulting on appropriate dosages for older people, look on the package insert for a section called "geriatric dosage." If such a section is not present, the old guideline of "start low, go slow" may hold true. More studies are needed to establish recommended geriatric dosages. Recently, several good texts have been published that give practical guidelines on the use of medications in the elderly.

Drug Prescribing in the Elderly, by Harrison Bloom and Elizabeth Schlom. Raven Press, New York, 1993. 299 pages 32.00 (paper).

Geriatric Pharmacology, edited by Rubin Bressler and Michael D. Katz. McGraw Hill, Inc., New York, 1993. 689 pages 49.95 (paper).

Handbook of Prescribing Medications for Geriatric Patients, by Judith C. Ahronheim. Little, Brown and Company, Boston, MA, 1992. 465 pages 30.00 (paper).

BROAD-SPECTRUM ANTIBIOTIC USE IN THE ELDERLY

The development of antibiotics in the 1930s and 1940s played a large role in the increased life expectancy of the population. Regardless of these pharmaceutical advances, however, infectious diseases still persist. About 25 percent of all contacts between physicians and patients still involve problems related to infections (Butler et al., 1994). An additional challenge to physicians is the changing patterns of antimicrobial resistance.

Since the advent of the prospective payment system and diagnostic-related groups for Medicare reimbursement, patients are being dismissed from hospitals sooner in the course

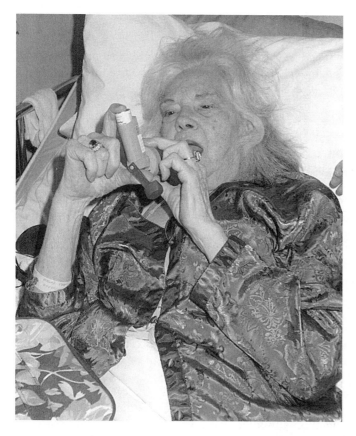

Figure 5-2   *Metered-dose inhalers.*

of illness. Many are sicker as they return home than were those in previous days who stayed in the hospital longer. Although early dismissal reduces hospital expense, microorganisms that used to be typical of hospital-acquired infections are now being seen in long-term care facilities. Additionally, long-term care patients with infections are not always transferred to acute care settings as was once the case. As a consequence, long-term care facilities are reporting more infections caused by penicillin-resistant *Streptococcus pneumoniae*, methicillin-resistant *Staphylococcus aureus* (MRSA), and vancomycin-resistant staphylococcus and *Enterococcus faecalis* (Butler et al., 1994). Providing safe and effective antibiotic therapy for community-acquired pneumonia and other infections is a goal of respiratory care practitioners nationwide (Sanders, 1994).

Beta-lactam antimicrobial agents, including penicillin and its derivatives, and extended-spectrum cephalosporins may be useful in treating pneumonia. The beta-lactam antibiotics are bactericidal. A complicating factor, however, is that bacterial resistance to beta-lactam antibiotics can occur through the action of an enzyme, beta-lactamase, which is produced by the bacteria (Rau, 1994). The emergence of beta-lactamase-producing bacteria parallels the history of antibiotic development.

When penicillin was first introduced in about 1940, virtually all strains of *Staphylococcus aureus* were susceptible to this beta-lactamase antibiotic. Today, more than 90 percent of *Staphylococcus aureus* worldwide is resistant to penicillin, ampicillin, and amoxicillin (Moellering, 1993).

Infections that currently are being seen in long-term care settings are increasingly difficult to diagnose and treat. Compounding the problem in long-term care facilities is that it is common for empirical therapy to be prescribed by the physician over the telephone. The physician may not see the patient for 1 or 2 weeks. Pathogens that possess antimicrobial resistance may be missed. The use of broad-spectrum antibiotics—ampicillin and cephalosporins—for empiric therapy may result in the creation of resistant micro-organisms. Some infections may be untreated, or undertreated, which may also play a role in breeding antimicrobial-resistant microorganisms. To counteract this evolving problem, sputum specimens for culture and sensitivity should be obtained so that identified bacteria can be treated with a more specific narrow-spectrum antibiotic.

Obtaining good sputum specimens, especially in elderly patients, may be difficult. Probably the best specimens—the ones that contain the least amount of epithelial cells—are obtained via nasotracheal suctioning. Narrowing and directing therapy to identifiable bacteria will minimize the emergent resistance of micro-organisms and maintain the effectiveness of broad-spectrum antibiotics for treatment of mixed infections (Butler et al., 1994).

Another class of agents now available for use are the beta-lactamase inhibitors. They inactivate the beta-lactamase enzymes before the enzymes can destroy the broad-spectrum antibiotic. Beta-lactam antibiotics, combined with beta-lactamase inhibitors, have a good safety record. These combined agents may be very useful in the treatment of community-acquired pneumonia or polymicrobial pneumonia.

A tried and true defense against the spread of micro-organisms is diligent handwashing! Unfortunately, the availability of antibiotics, the increased patient workload, the drive to be more conscious about time management, the use of gloves—which may create a false sense of security—the improved sanitary conditions surrounding today's health care providers, and the indestructible attitude of many practitioners have all been factors in reducing the vigilance to "old-fashioned" handwashing. Preventive management strategies such as handwashing, attention to patient hygiene—including skin, nails, and dentures—adherence to isolation policies and procedures, and attention to patient nutrition may all help reduce the spread of micro-organisms.

Broad-spectrum antibiotic therapy, when not deemed necessary, may be considered to be suboptimal care, because it increases the risks of superinfections and of introducing antimicrobial-resistant micro-organisms to the individuals or the surrounding environment (Butler et al., 1994).

MEDICAL GASES

Administration of medical gases is a common therapeutic modality delivered by respiratory care practitioners in both acute and long-term settings (Figure 5-3). As the basic fuel

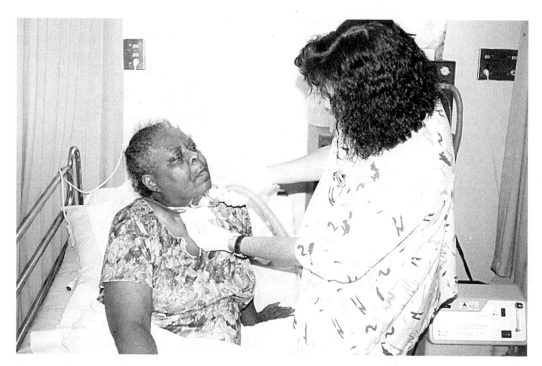

Figure 5-3 *Administration of medical gases.*

for aerobic life, oxygen is the most widely used therapeutic gas (Scanlan, Spearman, and Sheldon, 1990). Oxygen in excess of 21 percent delivered to a patient is considered to be a drug and requires a physician's prescription. Oxygen has, however, both beneficial and harmful effects. Respiratory care practitioners must be well versed in the goals and objectives of oxygen therapy as well as its hazards and limitations.

The beneficial effects of oxygen therapy in patients with chronic hypoxemia have been recognized for almost 60 years (O'Donahue, 1988). **Hypoxemia,** defined as an abnormally low arterial oxygen tension ($PaO_2 < 55$ mm Hg or $SpO_2 < 88\%$), may be caused by a variety of factors. Ultimately, hypoxemia leads to **hypoxia,** which is a deficiency of oxygen to the body tissues. Tissue hypoxia causes dysfunction of vital organs, which can lead to memory loss, impaired judgment, cardiac ischemia, and pulmonary hypertension (Tarpy and Farber, 1994).

Long-term oxygen therapy prolongs survival in patients with chronic obstructive pulmonary disease. Based on many studies and trials, this fact is widely accepted in the medical community. A study by the Nocturnal Oxygen Therapy Trial Group (1980) examined the efficacy of oxygen therapy on the survival of patients with COPD. The study established and justified the role of home supplemental oxygen for patients with COPD (Fletcher, 1994).

Due to physiological age-related changes in the lungs, older people usually experience some degree of hypoxemia. Documented hypoxemia, to an extreme, at rest will justify the prescription for oxygen therapy. Once the criteria for an oxygen prescription are met, a medical necessity form is filled out and an appropriate oxygen delivery system is selected. Without going into much more detail, in the final analysis, "Controlled clinical trials have clearly shown that oxygen has human benefit in terms of improved survival and quality of life" (Petty and Nett, 1983). Home oxygen therapy allows hospitalized patients to be discharged earlier, thus reducing the cost of medical care (O'Donahue, 1988). The forecast is for greater utilization of home oxygen in the United States and throughout the world.

ADVERSE DRUG REACTIONS

There are a number of potential problems with the use of medications in the elderly. "For the elderly, this may be the age of safe surgery and dangerous medicine" (Cohen, Lamy, and Fedder, 1984).

POLYPHARMACY

Overutilization of prescription and over-the-counter medications among the elderly is becoming increasingly recognized. Part of the problem is social. There is an expectation that when an individual visits the doctor, he or she will come away with a prescription. If not, the patient may be dissatisfied and "doctor shop." Also, some people may have a tendency to share medications with others, misuse current prescriptions, hoard old medications, and try them when they feel ill. Prescriptions may be filled at several different pharmacies, thus defeating the efforts of community pharmacists to evaluate and monitor drug regimens.

The other part of the problem is physical. Older people's kidneys and livers are less efficient in clearing medications from the body. Drug concentrations can build because they are not being metabolized and excreted. Older people also have proportionately less water in their bodies and proportionately higher ratios of fat to lean muscle mass. These factors may raise the concentration of certain medications in the body. Many older people move slowly, and too many get virtually no physical exercise. Activity level can increase metabolism; the lack of activity obviously must slow it down. Finally, older people are often smaller, their physical bulk is less, and medications given in normal adult dosages may, in effect, be overdoses.

Drugs should never be considered to be completely harmless, even if used correctly. Older people, for the most part, will not respond identically to the same therapeutic dosage of a given drug in comparison to younger adults or in comparison to other older adults. There are many factors involved in an elderly person's response to drug therapy that may change a normal dose to either a toxic or a subtherapeutic level. Either might result in an adverse drug reaction.

As defined by the World Health Organization, "Any response to a drug which is noxious and unintended and which occurs at doses used in man for prophylaxis, diagnosis or therapy" is termed an adverse drug reaction (Cohen, Lamy, and Fedder, 1984). There has been much discussion and little consensus over the years as to the precise, correct definition of adverse drug reactions. According to Reiss and Evans (1993), an adverse effect is one that a drug is capable of generating in addition to the intended effect. Drug reactions or effects have been further subclassified as to whether or not they are related to the pharmacologic effect of the drug.

SIDE EFFECTS

Side effects are the most common result of the pharmacologic effects of medications. Side effects occur due to a lack of specificity of action exhibited by most drugs, meaning that the drug acts not only on tissues for which it is intended but also with other tissues capable of responding to the administered drug.

As an example of side effects, nasal decongestants are sympathomimetic amines with primarily alpha-receptor action. The intended target is the alpha-receptor site. The response is vasoconstriction, which reduces the swelling of the nasal mucosa and reduces membrane congestion. One unintended target of nasal decongestants is the central nervous system, which when stimulated can result in side effects such as dizziness, drowsiness, and weakness.

Drug Toxicity.   Drug toxicity is an adverse side effect related to the dose of the drug administered. All drugs are capable of producing toxic effects. "Whenever you take a medicine, regardless of whether it is a prescription drug or non-prescription, there is a risk. The risk multiplies if you take more than one drug" (Cohen, Lamy, and Fedder, 1984).

A nationwide survey involving 36,000 nursing home residents in twenty-one states determined that an average of 5.15 routine medications per day and 3.23 as-needed (PRN) medications per day were taken by the residents (Simonson, 1994). A comparison of prescription medication usage in well elders and institutionalized elders revealed that well elders, ages 60 to 100, took an average of 3.9 different prescription medications per day. Institutionalized older people in the same age range averaged 6.0 prescriptions per day (Rice et al., 1994). In a study conducted at long-term care facilities, 32 percent of all the elderly patients received 8 or more different medications daily, and some received as many as 15 (Reiss and Evans, 1993). It is easy to see why drug toxicity and adverse drug reactions are such an issue when dealing with older people.

Less frequently encountered adverse drug reactions, such as allergic reactions and idiosyncratic reactions, are not the result of the drug's primarily pharmacological action but rather the response of the patient to the drug. Allergic reactions are the response of the patient's immune system to the presence of a drug, presupposing that the patient has previously come into contact (knowingly or unknowingly) with the drug or chemical and sensitization has occurred. Allergic responses to drugs may result in something as simple as a rash or hives or as serious as respiratory distress and circulatory collapse.

Idiosyncratic drug reactions are also abnormal responses to a drug or chemical. Unlike allergic reactions, which are dependent on prior sensitization, idiosyncratic reactions may occur with the patient's first exposure to the medication. An idiosyncratic reaction is an abnormal reactivity to a drug caused by a genetic difference between the reactive patient and nonreactive individuals (Reiss and Evans, 1993).

Regardless of the type of adverse drug reaction, in the elderly population it must be addressed. Adjustments in dosages, alteration of the dose schedule, drug discontinuance, or the addition of another drug are all steps that might be taken to alleviate the problem.

CASE STUDY

Esther was the pillar of her community at age 72. She was active in community group fundraisers, attended school sporting events, and could always be counted on to donate items for the hospital bazaar. The flower beds at her high-rise were beautiful, thanks to her loving care. She had been a widow for the past 10 years, but she continued to be active. Esther dismissed illness; she didn't have time to be sick. When any new ache or pain surfaced, she either had medication prescribed or purchased over-the-counter drugs to alleviate the symptoms. When she became quiet and withdrawn, her family started to worry. She angrily rejected their concerns, stating, "I'm just tired of doing everything." The reclusiveness became worse. Esther stayed in her apartment for days and became very agitated when her daughter tried to intervene. One afternoon, getting no response when she knocked on her mother's door, the daughter had the building supervisor open it, only to find her mother slumped in her chair, barely conscious.

After five days in the hospital and numerous tests, it was determined that Esther had over-medicated herself, almost to the point of death. Now, on carefully controlled medications, Esther can once again be seen at events around town. She is not as active as she once was, but everyone is glad to see her up and about.

A growing concern among the older population is **drug duplication,** which is the use of more than one drug with the same pharmacological properties for a problem or diagnosis usually treated with a single drug (Cooper, 1994). Concerns over drug duplication have even led to new terminology, which we mentioned at the beginning of this section—**polypharmacy.** Also known as *polymedicine,* this word describes the use of multiple drugs to treat chronic illnesses in older patients. In nursing homes, research indicates that the most common drug duplications are multiple laxatives, analgesics, NSAIDS, diuretics, hypnotics, antipsychotics, potassium supplements, vitamins, antacids, antinauseants, and antidiarrheals. Polypharmacy has been described as the principal drug safety issue among the aged (Cooper, 1994). Duplicate medications are often the result of older people seeing more than one physician. Patients often do not share this information with their doctor, and generally physicians do not think to ask if they are seeing another practitioner.

OVER-THE-COUNTER MEDICATIONS

Another related drug problem concerns the widespread usage of OTC preparations by older people. There are a significant number of OTC preparations available to patients with respiratory problems (Table 5-2).

Hospitalized patients rarely use nonprescription drugs. Once discharged, though, patients often resume self-medication with OTC preparations. Noninstitutionalized older adults who self-medicate are generally not monitored. The prevalence of chronic conditions

TABLE 5-2   Individual Ingredients Reviewed for Safety and Efficacy by FDA's OTC Drug Evaluation Division, Listed by Category of Respiratory Care

Antihistamines	Nasal Decongestants	Antitussives	Bronchodilators	Expectorants
Brompheniramine maleate (P)*	Allyl isothiocyanate (P)	Benzoate (IIS)	Aminophylline (IIS)	Ammonium chloride (P)
Chlorcyclizine HCl (P)*	Bornyl acetate (P)	**Camphor (I)***	Belladonna alkaloids (IISE)	Antimony potassium tartrate (IISE)
Chlorpheniramine maleate (P)*	Camphor (P)	Caramiphen edisylate (IIE)	**Ephedrine (I)***	Benzoin tincture compound (IIE)
Dexbrompheniramine maleate (P)*	Cedar leaf oil (P)	Carbetapentane citrate (IIE)	**Epinephrine (I)***	Calcium iodide (IISE)
Dexchlorpheniramine maleate (P)*	Creosote beechwood (P)	**Chlophedianol HCl (I)***	Eucalyptol (IIE)	Camphor (IIE)
Diphenhydramine HCl (P)*†	Ephedrine (P)	Cod liver oil (IIE)	Euphorbia pilulifera (IIE)	Chloroform (IISE)
Doxylamine succinate (P)	Eucalyptol (P)	**Codeine (I)***	Metaproterenol sulfate (IIS)	Creosote beechwood (IIE)
Methapyrilene (fumarate and HCl) (P)	Eucalyptus oil (P)	Creosote beechwood (IIE)	Methoxyphenamine HCl (IIE)	Eucalyptol HCl (IIE)
Phenindamine tartrate (P)*	Levomethamphetamine (P)	**Dextromethorphan (I)***	Pseudoephedrine HCl and sulfate (IIE)	Eucalyptus oil (IIE)
Pheniramine maleate (P)*	Menthol (P)	**Diphenhydramine HCl (IIE)*†‡**	**Racephedrine HCl (I)***	**Guaifenesin (I)***
Phenyltoloxamine dihydrogen citrate (P)	Naphazoline HCl (P)	Elm bark (IIE)	Theophylline (IIS)	Hydriodic acid syrup (IISE)
Promethazine HCl (P)	Oxymetazoline HCl (P)	Ethylmorphine HCl (IIE)		Iodized lime (IISE)
Pyrilamine maleate (P)*	Peppermint oil (P)	Eucalyptus oil (IIE)		Ipecac fluidextract and syrup (IIE)
Thenyldiamine HCl (P)	Phenylephrine HCl (P)	Hydrocodone bitartrate (IIS)		Menthol (IIE)
Thonzylamine HCl (P)*	Phenylpropanolamine bitartrate, HCl, & maleate (P)	**Menthol (lozenge & topical/inhalant) (I)***		Peppermint oil (IIE)
Triprolidine HCl (P)*	Propylhexedrine (P)	Noscapine (IIE)		Pine tar (IIE)
	Pseudoephedrine HCl and sulfate (P)	**Peppermint oil (I)***		Potassium guaiacolsol fonate (IIE)
	Thenyldiamine HCl (P)	Thymol (IIE)		Potassium iodide (IIE)
	Thymol (P)	Turpentine oil (oral) (IISE)		Sodium citrate (IIE)
	Turpentine oil (topical/inhalant) (P)	Turpentine oil (topical/inhalant) (IIE)		Squill (and squill extract) (IISE)
	Turpentine oil (oral) (P)			Terpin hydrate (IIE)
	Xylometazoline (P)			Tolu balsam (IIE)
				Turpentine oil (topical/inhalant) (IIE)
				Turpentine oil (oral) (IISE)
				White pine (IIE)

Note: List may not always include every form of ingredient (e.g., topical versus oral, multiple salts, etc.). Final rules on the safety and efficacy of these ingredients are not complete, with many ingredients likely to be ruled not generally recognized as safe and effective.

*Monographed as safe and effective.

†Includes diphenhydramine citrate.

‡The FDA proposed to include diphenhydramine as a monographed antitussive in an amendment proposed on 12/9/92 (57FR58378).

Key: (P) = pending, I = generally recognized as safe and effective and not misbranded, II = not generally recognized as safe and effective or misbranded, III = data insufficient for classification in II or III is indicated by S (safe) or E (effective).

Source: T. J. Witek and E. N. Schachter (1994). Pharmacology and therapeutics in respiratory care. Philadelphia: W. B. Saunders. Reprinted by permission.

in the aged, and the resultant symptoms of gastrointestinal disturbances, sleep complaints, chronic cough, arthritic aches and pains, and nervousness all lend themselves to attempted solutions through the use of OTCs. The cost of prescription drugs is another factor in some elderly patients' decisions to use the cheaper and more readily available OTC drugs. Since the mid-1970s, more than 600 products have been switched from prescription to OTC status, making nonprescription drug use even more convenient (Miller, 1996).

Common OTC drugs used by both well and institutionalized elderly people include vitamins, laxatives, analgesics, and antacids (Rice et al., 1994). The indiscriminate use of OTC drugs by older adults presents a challenge to all health care providers (Moore and Johnson, 1993). By themselves, OTC preparations taken judiciously usually are not a problem.

Even though OTC drugs can be obtained without a prescription, they are still capable of eliciting a toxic reaction. OTC drugs often contain the same active ingredient as prescription drugs, only at a lower dosage. The assumption is made that all consumers will read and follow the recommended dosage, as specified on the label. This may or may not happen. Some OTC drugs should not be used by patients with certain medical conditions.

Consider, for example, the case of a patient with chronic obstructive pulmonary disease and carbon dioxide retention. After a few restless nights, the patient decides to take an OTC sedative. The sedative effectively depresses the CNS and causes a slowing down of the respiratory rate. The decreased respiratory rate reduces the amount of carbon dioxide exhaled by the patient, further elevating the $PaCO_2$. Carbon dioxide narcosis and/or respiratory acidosis could be the result, putting the patient in a potentially life-threatening situation.

All over-the-counter drugs must be approved by the Food and Drug Administration (FDA). Regulation of OTC drugs, however, is not as stringent as the regulation of prescription drugs. In 1972, after years of relatively little control of nonprescription drugs, the FDA began reviewing OTC preparations (Reiss and Evans, 1993; Table 5-3). Instead of evaluating individual products, the FDA classified the active ingredients of the drugs by category of treatment—for example, as bronchodilators, expectorants, and so on (Witek and Schachter, 1994).

The problem in older patients arises when OTC medications and prescription drugs are taken simultaneously or inappropriately. Surveys of older people confirm that they take both OTC and prescriptions together on a routine basis. Their comments indicated that they saw no inherent danger in this practice. When asked about side effects, almost half said that they had drowsiness, headache, dizziness, and indigestion. When asked what they did about these side effects, 89 percent responded "nothing," stating that the symptoms of their illnesses were worse than the side effects of the medications (Moore and Johnson, 1993).

Where do respiratory care practitioners fit into this picture? As mentioned earlier, health care providers must serve as liaisons between the patient, pharmacist, and physician. A patient's drug history is vital to current medical management and must include both prescription and nonprescription drugs. The emergency room, however, where the first patient contact may take place, is not often the best setting to gather detailed, accurate drug history information. Home care therapists and visiting nurses are in an ideal position to question patients about their medication usage in a nonthreatening environment. Therapists assisting pulmonologists at outpatient clinics can gather drug histories along with the preappointment height, weight, and vital signs. Pulmonary function and sleep lab technologists may be able to provide important information to the physician about the patient's

TABLE 5-3 New Molecular Entities Approved as Respiratory Care Drugs During 1950–1990

NDA Number	Generic Name	Trade Name	Dosage Form	Applicant*	Pharmacologic Action	Classification†	Approval Date
13-601	Acetylcysteine	Mucomyst	Solution	Mead Johnson	Mucolytic	1-B	09-14-63
17-559	Albuterol	Proventil	Aerosol spray	Schering	Bronchodilator	1-B	05-01-81
19-402	Astemizole	Hismanal	Tablet	Janssen	Antihistamine	1-C	12-29-88
17-601	Azatadine maleate	Optimine	Tablet	Schering	Antihistamine	1-C	03-20-77
17-575	Beclomethasone dipropionate	Vanceril	Aerosol spray	Schering	Glucocorticoid	1-B	05-12-76
11-210	Benzonatate	Tessalon	Capsule	DuPont	Antitussive	—	02-10-58
18-770	Bitolterol mesylate	Tornalate	Aerosol spray	Winthrop-Breon	Bronchodilator	1-C	12-28-84
12-126	Chlophedianol hydrochloride	ULO	Syrup	Riker	Antitussive	—	11-03-60
17-661	Clemastine fumarate	Tavist	Tablet	Dorsey	Antihistamine	1-C	02-25-77
16-990	Cromolyn sodium	Intal	Capsule	Fisons	Antihistamine	—	06-20-73
12-649	Cyproheptadine hydrochloride	Periactin	Tablet	Merck Sharp & Dohme	Antihistamine	—	10-17-61
11-664	Dexamethasone	Decadron	Tablet	Merck Sharp & Dohme	Glucocorticoid	—	10-30-58
9-312	Dextromethorphan hydrobromide	Romilar	Syrup	Hoffman-La Roche	Antitussive	—	09-24-54
18-148	Flunisolide	Nasalide	Nasal solution	Syntex	Glucocorticoid	1-B	09-24-81
19-085	Ipratropium bromide	Atrovent	Inhaler	Boehringer Ingelheim	Anticholinergic	1-B	12-29-86
12-339	Isoetharine hydrochloride	Bronkosol	Solution for inhalation	Sterling	Bronchodilator	—	02-16-61
17-078	Isothipendyl hydrochloride	Theruhistin	Solution	Ayerst	Antihistamine	—	07-19-57
16-402	Metaproterenol sulfate	Alupent	Aerosol spray	Boehringer Ingelheim	Bronchodilator	—	07-31-73
19-193	Methacholine chloride	Provocholine	Inhaler	Hoffman-La Roche	Cholinergic	1-B	10-31-86
18-612	Nicotine resin complex	Nicorette	Gum	Merrill Dow	Ganglionic blocker	1-B	01-13-84
9-268	Oxtriphylline	Choledyl	Tablet	Warner-Lambert	Bronchodilator	—	03-03-54
19-009	Pirbuterol acetate	Exirel	Inhaler	Pfizer	Bronchodilator	1-C	12-30-86
9-987	Prednisolone	Delta-Cortef	Tablet	Upjohn	Glucocorticoid	—	06-21-55
9-766	Prednisone	Meticorten	Tablet	Schering	Glucocorticoid	—	02-21-55
18-859	Ribavirin	Virazole	Powder for reconstitution	Viratek	Antiviral	1-A	12-31-85
8-453	Succinylcholine chloride	Anectine	Injection	Burroughs Wellcome	Skeletal muscle relaxant	—	08-20-52
17-466	Terbutaline sulfate	Bricanyl	Injection	Merrill Dow	Bronchodilator	—	03-25-74
18-949	Terfenadine	Seldane	Tablet	Dow	Antihistamine	1-B	05-08-85
11-110	Triprolidine hydrochloride	Actidil	Tablet	Burroughs Wellcome	Antihistamine	—	04-14-58
11-919	Xylometazoline hydrochloride	Otrivin	Spray	Ciba	Adrenergic (vasoconstrictor)	—	10-22-59

Note: Excludes devices and those new molecular entities (NMEs) for which new drug application (NDA) was withdrawn prior to January 1, 1990.
*Applicant's name at the time of approval.
†NMEs approved before 1975 are not assigned therapeutic classifications. Chemical type: 1 = new molecular entity; 2 = new salt, ester, or derivative; 3 = new formulation; 4 = new combination; 5 = already marketed drug product; 6 = already marketed drug product by the same firm; 7 = already marketed drug product without an approved NDA. Therapeutic potential: A = important therapeutic gain; B = modest therapeutic gain; C = little or no therapeutic gain; AA = indicated for treatment of AIDS or HIV-related disease; V = designated orphan drug; E = developed, evaluated, or both, under special procedures for drugs intended to treat life-threatening and severely debilitating illnesses.
Source: T. J. Witek and E. N. Schachter (1994). Pharmacology and Therapeutics in Respiratory Care. Philadelphia: W. B. Saunders. Reprinted by permission.

drug use and related symptoms. Unless specifically asked, many elderly patients do not consider nonprescription drugs to be important enough to mention to the physician. Two concepts may be operative among some older patients: (1) "If it wasn't good for me, it wouldn't be sold in stores"; (2) "If my doctor didn't want me to take it, he or she would have told me."

COMPLIANCE TO DRUG THERAPY

Estimates of noncompliance in the ambulatory elderly vary from 40 percent to 80 percent (Cooper, 1994). These figures are disquieting, considering that in a recent report 40 percent of hospital admissions for drug-related illnesses in the elderly were associated with medication noncompliance (Col, Fanale, and Kronholm, 1990). One of the major issues in drug therapy for the elderly is lack of conformity to prescribed medication regimens. Patients generally adhere to medication schedules during hospitalization because health care professionals closely supervise their drug therapy. Shortly after discharge, though, for a variety of reasons, patients often discontinue taking drugs that were prescribed by the physician. Most geriatric patients continue to live in the community, outside of institutions. Therefore, most medications taken by older people are self-administered (Thorson and Thorson, 1979).

Compliance implies that the patient is taking the prescribed medication as directed at the correct time and at the proper dosage. Estimates of compliance among older patients are around fifty percent (Cooper, 1994). There can, of course, be variations and degrees of compliance, both intentional and non-intentional.

Noncompliance might be subclassified as either capricious or intelligent. Capricious noncompliance might be due to a misunderstanding or poor recollection of the health care professional's advice. Intelligent noncompliance describes behavior in which the patient fails to take medication because of a disagreement over what drug therapy is actually necessary. The practitioner should try to determine reasons for noncompliance. It might take some maturity on the part of the professional to realize that for a variety of reasons some older patients might be very much in touch with what is going on in their bodies. Those who have outlived three or four physicians, for example, might have a perspective on medicine and drugs that would be instructive to us all.

Geriatric patients living on their own and practicing self-medication have assumed responsibility for their own health care. Their pattern of drug compliance can be viewed as a continuum of total conformity to total nonconformity with a wide variety of behaviors in between. For the most part, patients intend to follow the prescribed pattern of drug administration. There are, of course, a number of factors that contribute to drug misuse or nonuse.

Comprehension of the directions given by the physician or other health care providers cannot always be assumed. Sick older people often have periods of confusion, and some older people are demented. Sometimes no directions or inadequate directions have been given. It is always a good idea to verify a patient's understanding of what medications should be taken, in what quantities, and at what times.

Some older people, especially those with arthritis, may have difficulty opening containers or manipulating devices. There are also sensory losses—difficulties with sight and hearing—that we have already discussed. Patients may have difficulty reading the label on a bottle of pills, and they may also have difficulty distinguishing between various tablets and capsules, especially those that are pale blue or green (Reiss and Evans, 1993). In addition to colors, the small size of many tablets and similarity in shape and dose form make it difficult for the patient to differentiate between pills. It may simply be difficult to pick them up or find them if they fall on the floor. Further, short-term memory lapses may make adherence to a drug regimen difficult. A patient in a doctor's office may be able to repeat a series of instructions but then not remember them an hour later. Dosage instructions should be written down in a type that is readable. Finally, patients taking a multitude of drugs may experience mental impairment and confusion as side effects (Ascione, 1994).

Drug Packaging. Elderly patients must be able to access the drug they are supposed to take. Many years ago, pharmaceutical manufacturers developed child-resistant containers, and more recently they have added tamperproof packaging. Although little doubt exists that these modifications have added a safety factor to medication usage, an artificial barrier has been created for older or compromised patients in accessing the medication. To address this problem, manufacturers of analgesics have now developed easy-open caps, which allow patients with arthritis unobstructed access to the medicine. Manufacturers of bronchodilators and other agents used in treating respiratory problems are also responding to the needs of the elderly or physically challenged patient populations.

In the past, patients with chronic obstructive lung disease that required at-home therapy were set up with paraphernalia that was at times almost unmanageable. Syringes or eyedroppers were needed to measure out the required milliliters of the bronchodilator, to mix with a measured amount of saline. Vision and dexterity problems made achieving uniform correct dosages almost impossible. Unit-dose, premixed, premeasured solutions now make nebulizer treatments more manageable. There have also been improvements in devices to maximize delivery of metered-dose inhalers, such as spacers, adaptors for patients with arthritis, and self-actuating inhalers that are triggered by the patient's inspiratory effort.

Finances. Finances may play a role in the compliance pattern of the patient, especially for those on a limited income. When a decision has to be made whether to purchase groceries or medications, food usually comes first. There is also a justifiable fear that after purchasing an expensive prescription the side effects encountered after three or four doses of the drug will render the medicine unusable. An ideal situation might be for the physician to send the older patient home with a few sample dosages of the desired pharmacological agent. If the patient tolerates the drug without noticeable adverse side effects, he or she might then be more likely to go ahead and purchase the prescribed drug, knowing that it would not be a waste of money. Another suggested intervention might be the substitution of a less expensive generic drug for the prescribed brand-name drug. Some caution is advised here, however.

Seventeen years after FDA approval is achieved, patents on brand-name drugs expire, and generic equivalents can be manufactured and sold by other pharmaceutical companies. To obtain FDA approval of a generic drug, manufacturers only need to show that it is safe and effective. The therapeutic equivalency between the brand-name drug and its generic equivalent is determined by the FDA. If attention is not given to the vehicle in which the medication is packaged, however, the drug may be chemically equivalent but therapeutically nonequivalent (Hogstel, 1994). Lamy has suggested that for some disease states and patient profiles generic equivalents should not be allowed (Cohen, Lamy, and Fedder, 1984).

Multiple Drug Regimens. The elderly as a group take more medications for a longer period of time than do younger age groups. They have a higher incidence of chronic disease, conditions that by definition do not lend themselves to a quick cure. Rather, the typical course of a chronic condition is management over time rather than an expectation of a cure. The increased numbers of drugs add to the complexity of the drug regimen, as older people are less likely to "go off" of a medication in a short period of time. Coupled with all of the other factors that lead to noncompliance, it is reasonable to assume that the complexity of the drug regimen could be inversely related to compliance. Older people who take multiple drugs may be prone to making errors in taking them (Hogstel, 1994). Unfortunately, this situation often leads to overmedication problems, especially taking repeat doses due to forgetfulness.

Psychosocial Characteristics. Psychosocial characteristics can also have a part in the use or misuse of medications. "If some is good, more is better" may be an attitude that becomes a complicating factor in appropriate drug delivery to the elderly. Taking too much of a drug could lead to unwanted side effects—stomach upset, sleeplessness or sleepiness, or tremor, for example. This situation could easily lead to noncompliant behavior such as not taking the drug at all in order to avoid side effects. Patients' perceptions of how well the drug is working, in the prescribed dosage, can lead to a variety of behaviors. The perception that a drug is prescribed as a prophylactic—need only be taken when in acute distress—can lead to numerous medical problems. Independent older people may adjust their dosage regimens simply in an effort to maintain control psychologically. Some older people do not like to take drugs at all, or they may have a swallowing problem manifested by a reluctance to take medications. Having to rely on chemical intervention is an admission of vulnerability and loss of independence. Others may like to take drugs and enjoy the attention that sick-role behavior brings (Thorson and Thorson, 1979).

Physicians are perceived as authority figures who command respect. Elderly females, especially those who were raised to be subservient and follow directions from men, may continue to consume medications even if no benefits are noticeable and the side effects are unpleasant. They might never presume to question the physician's authority. Those who seek out a physician as an authority figure might also resist going to a woman doctor.

IMPLICATIONS

Interventions may run the whole gamut of compliance issues, and these issues need to be addressed with every patient and by every caregiver. Because the majority of medications taken by older people are self-administered, health care practitioners have an important role in developing and implementing educational programs. Patients need to be informed on all aspects of their medications—what they are called, their indications, how often they need to be taken, at what time of the day, how many pills or capsules need to be taken at one time, and the possible side effects of each drug. Directions should be printed, in large type, as a reminder. There are many aids on the market to keep pills compartmentalized, as to day of the week and hours of the day. More important may be the follow-up and social contact with the patient to reinforce the importance of drug compliance. All members of the interdisciplinary team involved in the care of elderly patients have a responsibility to educate their patients and remain informed themselves on current medication practices. Only then can drug therapy in the elderly be effective.

SUMMARY

Drug therapy, however delivered, is the primary form of treatment for individuals with respiratory illnesses, regardless of age. The health care team's goal in geriatrics is to help the older adult walk a fairly fine line, minimizing disability and morbidity while avoiding misuse of medications. Correct use of the right medications has brought immeasurable relief to thousands of older respiratory patients.

Review Questions

1. List various reasons why some older patients are noncompliant in their medication regimens.
2. What symptoms might lead you to question the possibility of an adverse drug reaction?
3. What factors (e.g., sex, age, weight) play a role in your patients' pharmacological response to drugs?
4. Why are older adults more at risk for drug-related problems?
5. Describe a drug-related problem that you have personally encountered in patient care and explain how you handled the problem.

References

Ascione, F. (1994). Medication compliance in the elderly. *Generations, 18* (2), 28–30.

Beizer, J. L. (1994). Medications and the aging body: Alteration as a function of age. *Generations, 18* (2), 13–15.

Bennett, W. M. (1990). Geriatric pharmacokinetics and the kidney. *American Journal of Kidney Diseases, 16*, 283–288.

Bills, G. W., and Soderberg, R. C. (1994). *Principles of pharmacology for respiratory care.* Albany, NY: Delmar.

Bloom, H. G., and Schlom, E. A. (1993). *Drug prescribing for the elderly.* New York: Raven Press.

Butler, R. N., Cali, T. J., Louria, D. B., Parrott, M. A., et al. (1994). Rational use of broad-spectrum antibiotics in the elderly. *Geriatrics, 49* (supplement), S1–16.

Chalker, R. B., and Celli, B. R. (1993). Special considerations in the elderly patient. *Clinics in Chest Medicine, 14,* 437–442.

Cockroft, D. W., and Gault, M. H. (1976). Prediction of creatinine clearance from serum creatinine. *Nephron, 16,* 31–41.

Cohen, S. H., Lamy. P. P., and Fedder, D. O. (1984). *The medicated generation* (videotape). Baltimore: Department of Physical Therapy, School of Medicine, University of Maryland.

Col, N., Fanale, J. E., and Kronholm, P. (1990). The role of medication noncompliance and adverse drug reactions in hospitalizations of the elderly. *Archives of Internal Medicine, 150,* 841–845

Cooper, J. (1994). Drug-related problems in the elderly patient. *Generations, 18* (2), 19–21.

Cooper, J., Love, D. W., and Raffouel, P. R. (1982). Intentional prescription nonadherence (noncompliance) by the elderly. *Journal of the American Geriatric Society, 30,* 329–333.

Feldman, R. D., Limbird, L. E., Nadeau, J., Robertson, D., et al. (1984, March 29). Alterations in leukocyte beta-receptor affinity with aging. A potential explanation for altered beta-adrenergic sensitivity in the elderly. *New England Journal of Medicine, 310* (13), 815–819.

Fletcher, E. C. (1994). Controversial indications for long-term oxygen therapy. *Respiratory Care, 39,* 333–340.

Gleason, M. S. (1996). Pharmacologic issues in aging. *Critical Care Nursing Quarterly, 19* (2), 7–12.

Hogstel, M. O. (1994). *Nursing care of the older adult.* Albany, NY: Delmar.

Howder, C. L. (1992). *Cardiopulmonary pharmacology.* Baltimore: Williams and Wilkins.

Lamy, P. (1990). Clinical pharmacology. *Clinical geriatric medicine.* Philadelphia: W. B. Saunders.

Levitzky, M. G. (1991). *Pulmonary physiology.* New York: McGraw Hill.

McDonough, J. T. (Ed.) (1993). *Stedman's concise medical dictionary.* Baltimore: Williams and Williams.

Miller, C. A. (1994). Update on warfarin: Special considerations for the elderly. *Geriatric Nursing, 14,* 167–168.

Miller, C. A. (1996). Multiple choices in over-the-counter drugs. *Geriatric Nursing, 17* (5), 251–252.

Moellering, R. C. (1993). Meeting the challenges of beta-lactamases. *Journal of Antimicrobial Chemotherapy, 31* (suppl. A), 1–8.

Moore, J. F., and Johnson, J. E. (1993). Over-the-counter drug use by the rural elderly. *Geriatric Nursing, 14* (4), 190–191.

Nocturnal Oxygen Therapy Trial Group (1980). Continuous or nocturnal oxygen therapy in hypoxemic chronic obstructive lung disease. *Annals of Internal Medicine, 93,* 391–398.

O'Donahue, W. J. (1988). The future of home oxygen therapy. *Respiratory Care, 33,* 1125–1130.

Petty, T. L., and Nett, L. M. (1983). The history of long-term oxygen therapy. *Respiratory Care, 28,* 859–865.

Rau, J. L. (1994). *Respiratory care pharmacology.* St. Louis: Mosby.

Reiss, B. S., and Evans, M. E. (1993). *Pharmacological aspects of nursing care.* Albany, NY: Delmar.

Rice, P. A., Jensen, M., Lyons, M., and Murphy, F. (1994). Medications in well and institutionalized elders. *Geriatric Nursing, 15,* 216–218.

Sanders, C. V. (1994, March). New broad-spectrum agent addresses beta-lactam resistance. *Advance for Managers of Respiratory Therapy, 3* (2), 39–40.

Scanlan, C. L., Spearman, C. B., and Sheldon, R. L. (Eds.) (1990). *Egan's fundamentals of respiratory care.* St. Louis: C. V. Mosby.

Scarpace, P. J. (1988). Decrease receptor activation with age. *Journal of the American Geriatric Society, 36,* 1067–1071.

Simonson, W. (1994). Geriatric drug therapy: Who are the stakeholders? *Generations, 18* (2), 7–12.

Spratto, G. R., and Woods, A. L. (1993). *Nurse's drug reference.* Albany, NY: Delmar.

Tarpy, S. P., and Farber, H. W. (1994). Chronic lung disease: When to prescribe home oxygen. *Geriatrics, 49,* 27–33.

Thorson, J. A., and Thorson, J. R. (1979). Patient education and the older drug taker. *Journal of Drug Issues, 9,* 85–89.

Witek, T. J., and Schachter, E. N. (1994). *Pharmacology and therapeutics in respiratory care.* Philadelphia: W. B. Saunders.

CHAPTER SIX

ACUTE DISEASES
OF THE ELDERLY

———————— KEY TERMS ————————

ACE inhibitors
angioplasty
aspiration
atelectasis
bacteremia
cardiorhexis
chemoreceptor
community-acquired
  pneumonia
dysphagia

febrile
gastroesophageal reflux
  disease (GERD)
hiatal hernia
hospital-acquired
  pneumonia
hypochlorohydria
hypothalamus
hypothermia
immunodeficient

mechanoreceptor
osteoporosis
pulsus paradoxus
thrombus
tortuous
t-PA
Trendelenburg
venostasis

———————— LEARNING OBJECTIVES ————————

After completing this chapter, the reader should be able to:

1. Identify the leading causes of mortality from acute diseases in the elderly.
2. Discuss age-related changes that put older adults at risk for heart attacks.
3. Describe several therapeutic interventions in the treatment and management of a heart attack.
4. List the major acute respiratory diseases that are more prevalent in older adults.
5. Discuss similarities and differences in the diagnosis of asthma, emphysema, and chronic bronchitis.

6. Identify classes of pharmacological agents that are helpful in the treatment of acute exacerbations of chronic obstructive pulmonary disease (COPD).
7. Describe complications associated with trauma in older adults.
8. Discuss signs, symptoms, and treatment of hypothermia in the elderly.
9. Explain why postoperative complications may be more prevalent in the older adult patient.

INTRODUCTION

Losing one's health is an aspect associated with the aging process that is alarming to older adults. Health care providers deal with the results of poor health on a daily basis. Loss of functional ability is a frightening reality and is more noticeable among older patients.

Disease processes, whether they are chronic or acute, are not necessarily a function of age. It is the age-related physiological changes that put the elderly in a higher risk category. The geriatric population, like every other age group, is at risk for the unforeseen. Acute medical emergencies are not uncommon. Elderly people, however, have a reduced reserve capacity to cope with the stress that accompanies acute events.

This chapter discusses some of the more common cardiac and respiratory diagnoses. Circumstances that statistically show higher percentages of fatalities among older adults are also addressed.

As the population of older people increases, so does the number of hospital beds occupied by the elderly (Kern, 1991). More than 45 percent of intensive care unit beds are occupied by patients who are over 65 years old. More than 50 percent of all acute care admissions are for adults older than 75 (Fulmer and Walker, 1990). Emergency rooms also serve significant numbers of older people. Studies indicate that the top three reasons for older patients being seen in emergency rooms are (1) cardiovascular, (2) upper respiratory, and (3) falls and other injuries (Barnett, Harnett, and Bond, 1992). Heart attacks are the most frequent killer of older adults (Thorson, 1995). To understand the underlying causes of mortality due to heart attacks, the normal aging processes and age-related changes in the heart must be comprehended.

AGE-RELATED CARDIOVASCULAR CHANGES

The heart, like the rest of the body, undergoes gradual changes over time. In the absence of disease, however, the size of the heart remains essentially unchanged across the adult life span. An aged heart (Figure 6-1) may actually become somewhat smaller in later life as a result of decreased demand and reduced activity (Spence, 1989; Lamy, 1980).

However, because diseases of the heart and blood vessels are so common among older people, there is often some degree of cardiac hypertrophy. The vascular systems of older adults typically show some degree of atherosclerosis that affects the aorta, coronary arteries, and carotid artery (Hogstel, 1994a). Atherosclerotic changes also reduce the distensibility and elasticity of the arteries. Decreased arterial compliance, coupled with increased

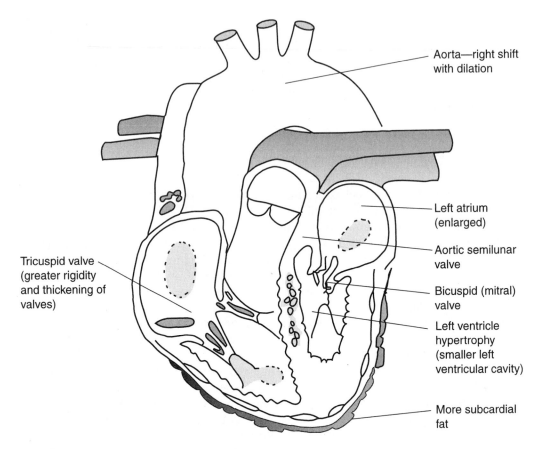

Aorta—right shift
with dilation

Left atrium
(enlarged)

Aortic semilunar
valve

Bicuspid (mitral)
valve

Left ventricle
hypertrophy
(smaller left
ventricular cavity)

More subcardial
fat

Tricuspid valve
(greater rigidity
and thickening of
valves)

Figure 6-1 *The aged heart.*

peripheral vascular resistance, results in a rise in systolic blood pressure and a slight in-crease in diastolic blood pressure (Needham, 1993), which puts an increased load on the left side of the heart, leading to left ventricular hypertrophy (Tierney, McPhee, and Papadakis, 1995). Other notable physiological changes include increased amounts of collagen and fat in the cardiac muscle and a thickening of the inside lining of the heart. Heart valves become thicker due to sclerosis and fibrosis. They also become more rigid. Calcification of the valves, especially the mitral valve, is not uncommon after age 60 (Spence, 1989). Aged hearts demonstrate a diminished stroke volume and reduced cardiac output.

When dealing with older patients it is important to understand that there is a decline in the heart's ability to handle stress. When stress is encountered, the heart rate and blood flow will increase, but the recovery time is much greater.

Structural changes in the conduction system of the heart may be related to the pro-longed recovery time. Infiltration of fat into the nodes and intraventricular bundle, a de-crease in the number of pacemaker cells, and sclerosis or fibrosis in the bundle of His may be factors in the heart's altered response to stress (Spence, 1989). Another hypothesis is that the extended recovery time is related to the catecholamine level in older adults, or to a reduction in response to catecholamines. Regardless of the cause, the cardiovascular system in older adults is usually compromised because of the effects of the aging process.

ACUTE CARDIOVASCULAR DIAGNOSES

Because older adults are two to three times more likely to suffer heart attacks than younger adults (Hellman and Williams, 1994), health care providers must be well educated and adequately prepared to effectively deal with cardiac problems in older patients. Heart disease is a major precursor to an acute heart attack. Heart attacks result from an acute blockage or an insufficient blood flow to the heart muscle. The region of the heart that is damaged from receiving little to no blood flow is said to be infarcted.

ACUTE MYOCARDIAL INFARCTION

A heart attack, more frequently referred to as an acute myocardial infarction (AMI), may cause death in a number of ways, depending on the location and severity of the damage. Myocardial infarction or myocardial ischemia may lead to cardiac arrest. Another cause of death may be extensive damage or destruction of the cardiac muscle cells themselves. The weakened cardiac muscle pumps a blood volume from the heart that is insufficient to sustain life. Death can be caused by a rupture of the weakened heart wall, also referred to as **cardiorhexis.** An infarction that affects the muscles of the ventricles could cause a delayed reaction. Diminished ventricular contraction would decrease cardiac output and reduce arterial pressure and blood flow. Concomitantly, the blood could accumulate in the veins, either pulmonary or systemic. For this reason, the patient who seems to be recovering after a heart attack could develop acute pulmonary congestion days after the infarction and die within a few hours (Spence, 1989).

Symptoms of Acute Myocardial Infarction. Symptoms that precede an impending AMI in older persons may be similar to those manifested in younger adults, but they may not be accompanied by severe pain. Deficiency in blood supply to the cardiac muscle, or ischemia, may not present with chest pain. In many cases, the substernal pain normally associated with heart attacks is not experienced by older persons (Hogstel, 1994a). Instead, the older patient will often have dyspnea, syncope, and exertional diaphoresis (Kern, 1991). Dyspnea, or shortness of breath, both at rest and with exertion, may be the most prevalent symptom. When dyspnea is the only sign noted, the patient may simply blame the symptoms on aging or other causes and not seek treatment (Needham, 1993). Acute myocardial infarction in the elderly may also present as an acute confusional state or as abdominal pain, weakness, and arrhythmias.

The older patient can pose some unique challenges. It becomes incumbent upon the health care professional to be alert for signs other than chest pain that may signify impending cardiac failure. Instead of classic chest pain, the elderly patient may present with confusion, syncope, stroke, vertigo, weakness, abdominal pain, persistent vomiting, or even cough. A sudden onset of intense dyspnea in advanced old age is often the most dominant symptom of AMI (Hazzard et al., 1994).

Treatment and Intervention.   After a diagnosis of AMI has been made, treatment and intervention measures are fairly standard—oxygen, hemodynamic monitoring, possible defibrillation, and pharmacologic intervention. Heart attack victims fortunate enough to reach the emergency room quickly may be treated with **t-PA** (tissue plasminogen activator) or other clot-dissolving drugs (Marieb, 1992). Other forms of medical management may include nitrates, lidocaine, calcium channel blockers, beta blockers, and angiotension-converting enzyme (ACE) inhibitors. When nitrates or nitroglycerine are used to prevent or treat angina, careful observation of blood pressure is required (Hogstel, 1994a). Lidocaine reduces primary ventricular fibrillation; however, the incidence of primary ventricular fibrillation is lower in those over age 65 (Hazzard et al., 1994). Because of reduced hepatic perfusion and drug metabolism in older adults, when lidocaine is used the loading dose and maintenance dose should be reduced.

Calcium blockers are generally well tolerated and potentially beneficial for elderly AMI patients. When calcium channel antagonists are used, however, the peripheral dilation achieved may also be accompanied by such side effects as edema, tachycardia, and orthostatic hypotension (Bloom and Schlom, 1993), giving added reason to monitor the patient closely. Beta blockers such as atenolol and metaprolol, which are beta$_1$ selective, may be preferable to nonselective beta blockers, especially among older people who have asthma or COPD. **ACE inhibitors,** such as captopril, enalapril, or lisinopril, may be beneficial in older AMI patients. The use of ACE inhibitors has been shown to reduce mortality and improve cardiac function.

Another commonly used pharmacologic agent—both a therapeutic and a prophylactic drug—is acetylsalicylic acid (ASA), aspirin. In a study population of over 2,000 patients with a clinical diagnosis of acute myocardial infarction, ASA was the most widely used of the proven therapies (Tsuyuki et al., 1994). "Take one aspirin every other day" is a common prescription for those patients prone to excessive clotting. Aspirin makes the blood platelets less sticky (Marieb, 1992).

If treatment requires a more aggressive course, there are quite a few options that may be considered. Coronary artery bypass grafting (CABG), which was first introduced in 1968, has been a common treatment for blocked coronary arteries or heart failure. In this procedure, a portion of an artery from another region of the body is grafted to provide an alternate route of blood circulation in the heart. Myocardial revascularization in the elderly has become routine, as evidenced by a fivefold increase in CABG surgeries from 1975 to 1990 in patients over age 65 (Brown, 1995; Fulmer and Walker, 1990).

Heart surgery in older adults is not without risk. Mortality rates after cardiac surgery increase for each decade of life after age 40 (Vaca, Lohmann, and Moskoff, 1994). On the upside, in patients over 65 years of age, data indicate that the operative mortality rate is only somewhere between 5 and 7 percent, with an 88 percent survival rate after 1 year (Brown, 1995). These statistics are a marked improvement over those of previous years.

Other invasive techniques that may be used to relieve blocked coronary arteries include balloon **angioplasty** and lasers. In angioplasty, an obstructed blood vessel may be dilated or reopened by threading a small catheter, followed by a balloon, into the obstructed vessel. By then inflating the balloon, the vessel is widened, the clot is compressed, and patency is restored. Although effective, the incidence of failed balloon catheter insertion due to **tortuous** or twisted, vessels and atherosclerosis may be higher in older patients. Laser beams that are transmitted through fine glass fibers may also be used to destroy clots (Spence, 1989).

Many older patients choose to treat their AMI passively or not at all. Advance directives and mutual decisions made with family and physicians may preclude some emergency care. These options are discussed more fully in Chapter 8.

CARDIAC REHABILITATION

If medical management of AMI includes invasive procedures, some type of reconditioning is usually necessary. Due to the nature and severity of cardiac surgery, many patients decrease their level of physical activity in the postoperative period. In actuality, some forms of cardiac rehabilitation exercise can be easily and safely accomplished by elderly patients. It is important that the nurses and therapists involved in rehabilitation programs are aware of the physiological changes in the cardiovascular and musculoskeletal systems of the elderly. There are some expected changes associated with the aging process that may affect exercise (Table 6-1).

After thorough evaluation of older cardiac rehab patients, realistic goals should be established based on their special needs and interests. Current research suggests that low-intensity exercise at the rate of 30 to 40 percent of heart rate reserve may be just as beneficial as high-intensity training at 60 to 70 percent of heart rate reserve (Hellman and Williams, 1994). It may even be superior, considering compliance and safety issues. Postoperative CABG patients should avoid arm exercises until their incision is healed, but after that reconditioning is important. Exercises such as walking, armchair aerobics, floor exercises, cycling and even mild calisthenics may be very beneficial.

TABLE 6-1 Expected Changes Associated with Aging That May Affect Exercise

---

Reduction in maximal aerobic power
Reduction in cardiovascular reserve (primarily due to lower maximal heart rate)
Reduction in elasticity of the peripheral vasculature
Reduction in musculoskeletal strength
Reduction in elasticity of connective tissue
Reduction in musculoskeletal flexibility
Increasing prevalence of symptomatic and asymptomatic coronary artery disease
Increasing prevalence of chronic diseases such as hypertension, diabetes mellitus,
    degenerative bone and joint diseases, and malnutrition

Source: *Esther Hellman and Mark Williams (1994). Outpatient cardiac rehabilitation in elderly patients.* Heart and Lung, 23, *506–511.*

Rehabilitation programs should be tailored to individuals. Elderly patients with heart disease usually respond favorably to low-intensity training when they gradually increase the frequency and duration of exercises. Progress of the older patient may be slower, but there will usually be improvement in the patient's overall functional abilities after participating in a cardiac rehab program.

Although heart disease remains the leading cause of death for persons 65 and older, the death rate has been declining considerably among all adult age groups (Barrow, 1989). Changes in diet, modifications in social behavior (smoking and alcohol consumption), and an increased interest and participation in exercise programs have all been factors in reducing death rates from heart attacks. Decreased cardiac disability, the promotion of personal independence, and an elevated level of self-esteem and life satisfaction are all achievable among the aged (Hellman and Williams, 1994).

ACUTE RESPIRATORY DIAGNOSES

Upper respiratory problems are the second-largest causative factor in visits to emergency rooms by older adults. Upper respiratory diagnoses, although not all technically upper respiratory, encompass a wide range of illnesses. Included may be anything from acute exacerbations of COPD, to pneumonia, to aspiration of a foreign object—with a myriad of reasons in between. To narrow the focus, this section highlights some of the more common acute respiratory abnormalities that require immediate treatment.

ACUTE EXACERBATIONS OF COPD

An acute exacerbation of asthma, chronic bronchitis, or emphysema can be frightening and life-threatening. Chronic bronchitis and emphysema are both more common in older adults and frequently occur together. Dyspnea is probably the most common presenting symptom. Other physical signs noted upon hospital admission are agitation, use of accessory muscles of inspiration, and alterations in mental status. During a severe attack of bronchospasm, there may be an increase in the magnitude of **pulsus paradoxus,** or the change in blood pressure with the different phases of respiration (Dantzker, MacIntyre, and Bakow, 1995). Hypoxemia in most of these patients is already present, with or without carbon dioxide retention. An acute exacerbation is very likely the result of an event that worsened the patient's existing hypoxemia.

During an acute phase, it may be difficult to distinguish among asthma, chronic bronchitis, and emphysema. The use—or perhaps overuse—of the term *COPD* to classify all of these diseases may not be helpful. Although the treatments may be similar, the therapeutic regimen for each disease may be different enough to warrant a specific diagnosis.

Asthma patients generally present with dyspnea and a wheeze. The wheeze is occasionally present in the patient with chronic bronchitis, but usually absent in the patient with emphysema. A productive cough is more indicative of chronic bronchitis. Asthmatics often present with a cough, but it is usually nonproductive. Emphysematous patients rarely cough. Older patients with emphysema often trap air in the lung periphery at the end of exhalation. Over time, the loss of elasticity of lung tissue and hyperinflation lead to a "barrel chest" appearance. This barrel chest can be helpful in distinguishing emphysema from asthma and chronic bronchitis (Dantzker, MacIntyre, and Bakow, 1995). The challenge comes in diagnosing the patient with components of all three diseases.

CASE STUDY

John was admitted to the intensive care unit at 4:20 A.M. in acute respiratory distress. ABGs on room air revealed the following: pH = 7.25, $PaCO_2$ = 86, PaO_2 = 54, HCO_3 = 36. At 62 years of age, John had often been a patient at this small community hospital. A diagnosis of COPD and CHF (congestive heart failure) years before had convinced him to cut back on his smoking, but he did not quit. A few weeks earlier, John's sister-in-law had been in a bad accident. He'd had trouble sleeping, so he asked the doctor to give him "something for his nerves." John was already taking nebulized isoetharine hydrochloride treatments at home, along with theophylline, furosemide, prednisone, ampicillin, guaifenesin, digoxin, amitriptyline hydrochloride, and phenylephrine hydrochloride. The physician was hesitant to add any new drugs to John's therapeutic regimen. He assured John that he just needed to stop worrying about things he couldn't control and focus more on keeping himself healthy. Earlier that evening, prior to coming to the hospital, John had a few beers. When he couldn't get to sleep, he'd also taken an over-the-counter sleeping pill.

1. Was it one factor or a combination of factors that led to John's hospitalization?
2. If you had been on duty when John was admitted, what course of treatment would you have recommended?

Treatment. Initial treatment usually consists of low-flow oxygen and lab work, including arterial blood gases, to determine the severity of the problem. Oxygen not only reduces the work of breathing but also reduces the work of the heart. Fast-acting beta-agonists are the drugs of choice in treating an acute exacerbation. Aerosolized sympathomimetics such as albuterol or metaproterenol have a rapid onset of action. Because of fewer side effects, albuterol is the aerosol of choice among elderly and/or cardiac patients (Bloom and Schlom, 1993). Relaxation of the bronchial smooth muscle helps relieve the bronchospasm. If the patient is able to perform an expiratory maneuver, measurement of the pre- and postbronchodilator peak flow is useful. If the patient has asthma or a reversible component, the expiratory flows will be greatly improved after a bronchodilator treatment. Another class of medications that may be aerosolized are anticholinergics. Ipratropium bromide effectively blocks vagally mediated reflex bronchoconstriction and is often used in the treatment of acute asthma. Atropine is also an effective anticholinergic agent, but has systemic side effects. Because of potential adverse side effects, caution is indicated in using anticholinergics in adults over age 70.

Corticosteroids are effective anti-inflammatory agents. How and why they improve lung function in patients with pulmonary disease is not precisely understood, but they are beneficial. Often, older patients will already be on inhaled steroids, prescribed for their pulmonary diagnosis. Patients who develop an acute exacerbation of COPD while on inhaled steroids might benefit from a trial of systemic steroids (Bloom and Schlom, 1993). Xanthines are another class of drugs that may be useful in acute exacerbations. Their precise mechanism in producing bronchodilation is also not well understood. The improvement in airflow may be more a factor of strengthened diaphragmatic contractility and central respiratory stimulation than bronchodilation.

Regardless of the drug or drugs used to reverse the bronchospastic airway, once the crisis is over management must be directed at treating the initial cause of the exacerbation. Unfortunately, not all older adults who enter the emergency room in acute exacerbation can be turned around. If the patient's condition gradually worsens and respiratory failure is impending, assisted ventilation may be recommended and/or instituted.

RESPIRATORY FAILURE

Regardless of the etiology, respiratory failure results in inefficient pulmonary gas exchange, as evidenced by abnormal blood gases. Generally accepted conditions that are present—collectively or individually—when a patient is diagnosed as being in respiratory failure are (Eubanks and Bone, 1990):

- Acute dyspnea
- PaO_2 < 50 torr on room air
- $PaCO_2$ > 50 torr
- pH < 7.35

The most common reasons that older patients present to the emergency room in acute respiratory failure are complications involving obstructive or restrictive lung diseases, pneumonia, and pulmonary edema. Ventilation/perfusion abnormalities or shunt mechanisms are usually the cause of hypoxemia in these pulmonary disorders.

Immediate Treatment. Immediate treatment consists of reversing the hypoxemia with oxygen therapy and then treating the patient based on the differential diagnosis. If hypercapnia is present and results in respiratory acidosis, aggressive treatment is necessary. Hyperinflation modalities (intermittent positive pressure breathing or continuous positive airway pressure) may be considered as therapeutic interventions. A more frequent treatment for respiratory failure is intubation followed by mechanical ventilation.

The decision to initiate mechanical ventilation in cases of respiratory failure in older adults is sometimes difficult. Ideally, such decisions are jointly made by the physician, spouse, and other family members. Age alone should not be a determining factor. The presence of an end-stage terminal illness versus an acute, reversible process is one obvious consideration. Factored into the decision-making process should also be a discussion concerning the likely benefits and/or complications associated with long-term ventilation. The whole issue of informed consent leads to ethical and legal questions. In an emergency situation, is there time to give adequate information and assure competence of the patient? If a surrogate is involved, is that person indeed looking out for the patient's best interests? Withholding or initiating ventilator therapy is covered in greater detail in Chapter 8.

ASTHMA

As previously discussed, asthma is normally classified as a chronic lung disease. Status asthmaticus, however, is an acute, life-threatening attack of asthma, in which the degree of airway obstruction is severe to begin with, and increases in severity with little or no response to the usual treatments. Acute, life-threatening attacks of asthma do occur as frequently in the elderly as in younger asthmatics (Dantzker, MacIntyre, and Bakow, 1995). According to the *Guidelines for the Diagnosis and Management of Asthma,* a 1991 publication developed by the National Heart, Lung, and Blood Institute and the National Asthma Education Program, studies indicate that the increase in asthma mortality throughout the world is more marked in older (greater than 55 years) patients with asthma.

Because of diagnostic difficulties, the precise cause of severe airflow obstruction is sometimes difficult to identify. Older patients with asthma may also have some degree of cardiac disease. The clinical signs of tachycardia, wheezing, and pulsus paradoxus during inspiration may occur in a patient with left ventricular failure (Dantzker, MacIntyre, and Bakow, 1995) or in a patient with asthma. The differential diagnosis must be made carefully to determine if the cause of wheezing is cardiac or pulmonary.

A precipitating factor in severe asthma in the elderly may be the presence of comorbid conditions. There is nothing that excludes patients from having COPD as a result of smoking and also having asthma (Kyes, 1994). Some patients have asthma and coronary artery disease. The presence of a chronic disease will diminish the body's ability to respond to an acute situation. In older asthmatics with heart disease, hypoxemia must be monitored closely. Patients with coronary artery disease, suffering an acute asthma attack with associated hypoxemia, could also sustain cardiac damage or rhythm disturbances.

Arthritis often coexists with asthma (O'Brien-Ladner, 1994). Aspirin and NSAIDS used in the treatment of arthritis could aggravate asthma, leading to bronchospasm. Elderly asthmatic patients with glaucoma or cataracts are at risk when the beta-blocker, timolol, an ophthalmic preparation to reduce intraocular pressure, is prescribed. The *Journal of Family Practice* has reported a case of timolol eyedrop-induced fatal bronchospasm in a 70-year-old asthmatic patient hospitalized for cataract extraction. Many ophthalmologists have now switched to betaxolol, a potent and selective beta-adrenergic blocking agent (Odeh, Oliven, and Bassan, 1991). Although several studies have demonstrated that topically applied betaxolol has no significant effect on the respiratory system, patients with asthma should be monitored closely for undesirable side effects when the use of any beta-blocker is necessary.

Unfortunately, it is not just the comorbid conditions that put older patients with asthma at a higher risk for acute asthmatic episodes. Medications prescribed to treat other geriatric medical problems such as glaucoma and arthritis, as well as dosage forms, pose additional dilemmas for the elderly. There are a wide variety of drugs now available in metered-dose inhaler (MDI) form for asthmatic patients. These drugs may be short-acting, beta$_2$-agonists (1 to 6 hours in duration), long-acting beta$_2$-agonists (8 to 12 hours in duration), corticosteroids, anticholinergics, or anti-inflammatory agents. A review of Rau's *Respiratory Care Drug Reference* (1997) reveals that there are at least sixteen different FDA-approved MDIs that may be prescribed by a physician to treat asthma, or purchased as OTC inhalers available at the local drugstore. When in acute distress, older people may become confused and use the wrong MDI. When immediate relief is needed, using the inappropriate MDI may lead to a false sense of security, and much-needed medical intervention may be delayed. It has also been suggested that older patients have a reduced awareness of moderate airway obstruction, thus postponing self-referral for medical help.

Treatment. Regardless of the cause, the main goals when treating the elderly patient with asthma in the emergency room are to correct hypoxemia and rapidly relieve the airflow obstruction. Hypoxemia can be treated initially with low-flow oxygen and monitored by arterial blood gases and oximetry. Airflow obstruction caused by bronchospasm, mucosal edema, and/or excessive secretions is initially treated by administering rapid-acting beta$_2$-agonists, with systemic steroids often following. According to Burrows (cited in Kyes, 1994), prescribing oral steroids to elderly patients is not as common as it once was. Unfortunately, it was difficult to get the patients off the steroids because patients liked the way they felt on steroids regardless of the drug's effectiveness. Inhaled steroids provide treatment for asthma without as many adverse side effects. Acute asthma, however, remains a challenge. When patients present with an acute exacerbation, the therapy continues to be high doses of oral steroids, tapered down to maintenance doses and then a gradual switch to inhaled steroids.

Always be aware of the possibility that the wheezes heard may be cardiac, not asthma, or that both conditions may coexist. In a patient with left ventricular failure, high-dose steroid therapy may precipitate cardiac failure (Dantzker, MacIntyre, and Bakow, 1995). In this situation, hemodynamic monitoring with a Swan-Ganz catheter may be advisable. Older people are also more prone to steroid psychosis when treated with high doses of steroids. When possible, maximal use of oral, parenteral, and aerosolized bronchodilators is desirable.

PULMONARY EDEMA

Pulmonary edema is the excessive movement of fluid from the pulmonary vessels through the interstitium and into the air spaces of the lungs (Des Jardins and Burton, 1995). Patients with acute pulmonary edema normally present with severe respiratory distress, hypoxemia, and tachypnea. Because pulmonary edema can be a life-threatening condition, medical management must be instituted rapidly. Appropriate treatment of pulmonary edema depends on identification of the cause (Scanlan, Spearman, and Sheldon, 1995).

Pulmonary edema may be classified as cardiogenic or noncardiogenic. Cardiogenic pulmonary edema is caused by elevated capillary hydrostatic pressures that are excessive enough to result in a fluid leakage into the interstitium. Once the interstitium is flooded, the fluid will cross the alveolar–capillary membrane and leak into the alveoli.

Why is there an increased incidence of pulmonary edema in older people? Refer again to the age-related physiological changes in the cardiopulmonary system. Left ventricular failure is the most common cause of cardiogenic pulmonary edema (Scanlan, Spearman, and Sheldon, 1995). Left ventricular hypertrophy, resulting in part from increased systemic vascular resistance, is often noted in older people. Years of distension and excessive work can cause the cardiac fibers to lose some strength, which in turn results in a reduced left ventricular cardiac output. Because the left ventricle does not empty completely, blood backs up and accumulates in the pulmonary vessels. This fluid backup increases capillary pressures, resulting in pulmonary edema. Other causes of cardiogenic pulmonary edema that are more prevalent in the elderly may be arrhythmias, mitral stenosis, renal failure, systemic hypertension, and myocardial infarctions.

Increased capillary permeability as a result of infections and inflammation may cause noncardiogenic pulmonary edema. Alterations in alveolar surfactant may contribute to the increased capillary permeability. Increased fluid in the alveoli caused by massive capillary leakage in the presence of normal hydrostatic pressures results in acute respiratory distress.

Treatment and Management. Effective treatment of patients presenting with pulmonary edema requires accurate assessment. Adequate ventilation must be achieved as quickly as possible. Hypoxemia, usually associated with pulmonary edema, necessitates the use of oxygen therapy. Left ventricular failure may be treated with drugs that stimulate heart muscle contraction and thus increase cardiac output. Systemic hypertension may be reduced with direct-acting vasodilators. Morphine sulfate, in addition to relieving anxiety, increases venous capacitance, thus decreasing venous return and decreasing atrial pressure (Dantzker, MacIntyre, and Bakow, 1995). *One note of caution:* In elderly individuals a normal therapeutic dose of morphine can be fatal (Bills and Soderberg, 1994). Diuretics may be used with caution to promote fluid excretion.

In addition to pharmacologic agents, hyperinflation therapy is often prescribed to offset the fluid accumulation in the alveoli and reverse the **atelectasis** associated with pulmonary edema (Des Jardins and Burton, 1995). Mechanical ventilation may be instituted in an effort to assure adequate ventilation and oxygenation. In recent years, an increasing number of authors have reported their experience in the management of acute and subacute respiratory failure with noninvasive mechanical ventilation by nasal mask (Chesi et al., 1994). The noninvasive mechanical ventilation was well tolerated by older patients, but it did not alter the long-term prognosis of patients with preexisting left ventricular failure.

Once the acute phase of pulmonary edema has been treated, the underlying cause must be determined in an effort to prevent future occurrences.

PNEUMONIA

Pneumonia and influenza, added together, are the fourth-leading cause of death for people 65 and older (Sobol and Fleming, 1994). Pneumonia is an inflammatory process that primarily affects the gas exchange units of the lungs (Des Jardins and Burton, 1995).

Older adults are at an increased risk for pneumonia, as well as other infectious diseases, because of their depressed immune systems. Until proven otherwise, all older persons must be considered **immunodeficient** (Louria, 1994). Improper nutrition may well be a factor that affects older people's ability to fight infection. Age-related loss of elasticity in the lung tissue increases the risk for developing pneumonia. Decreased elasticity of lung tissue and a gradual loss of flexibility of the rib cage diminishes the overall depth of ventilation. Even though there is a compensatory increase in the respiratory rate, this diminished depth of breathing may increase the risk of developing respiratory problems, including pneumonia, in the aged (Hogstel, 1994a).

Although there are many etiological reasons, the leading causative agents of pneumonia are viral and bacterial. Taking this one step further, pneumonia can also be classified in the aged as community acquired, hospital acquired, and nursing home acquired.

Community-Acquired Pneumonia. **Community-acquired pneumonia** occurs in individuals who are usually ambulatory and living in a noninstitutional environment (Butler, 1994). Two major organisms that cause community-acquired pneumonia are pneumococcus and *Haemophilus influenzae*. About 20 to 30 percent of patients with pneumococcal pneumonia develop **bacteremia,** or bacteria in the blood. At least 20 percent of the patients diagnosed with bacteremia die from it.

Hospital-Acquired Pneumonia. **Hospital-acquired pneumonia** is a more complex problem. Anaerobes and gram-negative organisms are more likely to be involved (Pearl, 1994). The relationship between increased mortality, advanced age, and gram-negative pneumonia is well established. In patients older than 40 who develop gram-negative pneumonia, mortality may be as high as 70 percent (Dantzker, MacIntyre, and Bakow, 1995).

Pneumonia acquired in a nursing home or long-term-care facility may be caused by either bacteria or a virus, but the most probable cause of pneumonia in this setting is aspiration.

Aspiration Pneumonia. **Aspiration** is the inhalation of foreign material into the airway. Aspiration may lead to acute problems in any age group, but there are characteristics common to the elderly that put them at greater risk.

An obvious factor among some older adults is the lack of teeth and the problem of loose-fitting dentures. The lack of opposing molars to adequately chew food could result in an attempt to swallow larger portions of food. The gag reflex is less effective in the elderly, increasing the danger of choking (Needham, 1993). There is also a decline in salivary flow that accompanies aging, thus making swallowing more difficult.

Dysphagia, or difficulty in swallowing, whether real or perceived, may precipitate aspiration. Dysphagia may have numerous underlying causes. A dry mouth, directly related to the decline in salivary flow, or indirectly related to dehydration, will impair the ability to swallow. Certain drugs such as antidepressants, anticonvulsants, and amphetamines can cause a dry mouth (Hogstel, 1994a). The loss of muscle tone, commonly accepted as an age-related physiological change, may result in reduced esophageal motility. Other underlying causes of dysphagia may be neurological in nature or may be the result of a stroke. Nutrition may play a role in the development of dysphagia. Patients with Alzheimer's disease often have nutritional deficiencies, among them a lack of vitamin B_{12} (Miziniak, 1994). A B_{12} deficiency, or failure to absorb vitamin B_{12}, is also common to pernicious anemia. One symptom of pernicious anemia is dysphagia. Dryness and thirst are also common symptoms among diabetics. Added to this situation is the fact that esophageal peristalsis slows and the esophageal sphincter is less efficient in the elderly, which may cause delayed entry of food into the stomach and may increase the risk of aspiration (Needham, 1993).

The occurrence of **hiatal hernia,** a protrusion of a portion of the stomach through the esophageal hiatus of the diaphragm, increases rapidly as aging progresses (Hogstel, 1994a).

Most hiatal hernias are asymptomatic and do not require treatment. Others may be problematic but still produce no symptoms. One reason for this is the decremental change in the gastric mucosa, which leads to a reduction in the production of hydrochloric acid. A recent study demonstrated that in one-third of older subjects the production of gastric acid had decreased as a result of atrophic gastritis, which neutralizes gastric acid (Raiha, Ivaska, and Sourander 1992). Health care providers need to be alert and provide prompt attention when a patient complains of discomfort associated with hiatal hernia. Regurgitation and aspiration of gastric contents can lead to serious problems such as pneumonia.

Gastroesophageal reflux disease (GERD), in which there is a reflux of the stomach contents into the esophagus, is not necessarily more common among older people, but it may cause more damage. The reduction of hydrochloric acid production, **hypochlorohydria,** increases the pH of gastric acid, which in turn reduces the pain associated with reflux. Because little or no pain is felt when reflux occurs, the patient may not be aware that there is a problem. Pulmonary damage caused by GERD is assumed to appear more often in elderly patients because they have suffered from the disorder for many years. Respiratory function in elderly patients with this condition has been studied (Raiha, Ivaska, and Sourander, 1992). A restrictive pulmonary defect based on spirometry results was associated with GERD in the aged.

Aspiration pneumonia may be caused by the aspiration of gastric contents. It may result in the lungs being infected with several organisms, some of which are not normally pathogenic (Levitzky, Cairo, and Hall, 1990). The physiologic response to gastric acid aspiration usually starts with a rapid development of atelectasis. This results in a decreased arterial oxygen tension (PaO_2), followed by an influx of fluid into the lungs (Dantzker, MacIntrye, and Bakow, 1995). Bacterial infection may or may not be a complicating factor. The aspiration of oropharyngeal microbes may result in aspiration pneumonia, especially if the patient has any periodontal disease. Aspiration of oropharyngeal contents during sleep is not uncommon in healthy adults. Elderly patients with reduced levels of consciousness are much more likely to aspirate oropharyngeal bacteria during sleep, especially if they sleep predominantly in a supine position.

The diagnosis of aspiration pneumonia can be serious and is often fatal. Unfortunately, it is not an uncommon diagnosis, particularly in postoperative critical-care supine patients (Pearl, 1994). Mortality rates from aspiration pneumonia increase when conditions such as bacterial pneumonia and/or acute respiratory distress syndrome (ARDS) develop in patients who aspirate acidic gastric contents.

Aspiration is probably the leading cause of pneumonia among patients residing in long-term-care facilities (Pearl, 1994). The presence of gastric or nasogastric tubes used to deliver nutritional support increases the risk of aspiration and resultant aspiration pneumonia. Therapists have long been taught that the presence of a cuffed artificial airway will protect the lower airway from aspiration. According to Pearl, endotracheal tubes, at best, probably provide only about 75 percent protection to the patient's airway. Secretions that pool on top of the cuff, which cannot be suctioned effectively, can be aspirated.

Data indicate that prolonged endotracheal intubation (>24 hours) impairs the swallowing reflex (deLarminat et al., 1995). Intensive care patients may demonstrate dysfunction of the swallowing reflex for as long as 7 days postextubation. Factors involved in the delayed swallowing reflex may be residual effects of sedative drugs or even the presence of naso-gastric tubes. The alteration of **chemoreceptors** and **mechanoreceptors** located in the pharyngeal and laryngeal mucosa, associated with prolonged contact of the artificial air-way, may play a role in delayed swallowing. Whatever the cause, this phenomenon of an impaired swallowing reflex could contribute to the incidence of aspiration pneumonia after extubation (deLarminat et al., 1995).

Intervention. In dealing with the problem of aspiration, perhaps the best defense is a good offense, which starts with education. Knowledge of the factors that lead to aspiration can assist health care providers in carrying out simple precautionary measures. There are many modifications that can be made, without major expense to the family or medical facility, to decrease the risk of aspiration. Suggested interventions to prevent or reduce the incidence of aspiration include:

1. Avoid bedtime snacks and a reclining position for at least an hour after meals in patients with known hiatal hernia or GERD. Consider elevating the head of the bed on blocks.
2. Allow adequate time for meals and assist the patient if necessary. A "hurry up and eat" mode will only cause problems.
3. When performing postural drainage or chest physiotherapy on a patient with a feeding tube in place, put feeding on hold for 20 to 30 minutes before putting the patient in the **Trendelenburg** (head down) position.
4. When performing postural drainage or chest physiotherapy on a patient with a regular diet, try scheduling treatments to fall 1 hour or more after meals.
5. When performing postural drainage or chest physiotherapy on a mechanically ventilated patient, be careful not to let tubing condensate drain back into the endotracheal tube.
6. Turn the head of an unconscious patient to the side to prevent aspiration. A mild Trendelenburg position will also promote drainage in a cephalad direction (Dantzker, MacIntyre, and Bakow, 1995).
7. Check the patency and function of nasogastric tubes at regularly scheduled intervals.
8. Monitor patients with endotracheal or tracheostomy tubes in place. Use sterile suctioning techniques as frequently as necessary.
9. Monitor patients after extubation for impaired swallowing reflexes.

Treatment and Prevention. Treatment guidelines for the elderly patient are governed by the infective agent and/or causative factor. The incidence of community-acquired pneumonia, caused most often by pneumococcus, can be reduced by a simple vaccination. The shot, which is covered by Medicare, can be a lifesaver (Thorson, 1995). Unfortunately, the vaccination is underused because of public resistance and cost reimbursement difficulties (Pearl, 1994). Only 14 percent of those 65 and older were immunized against pneumococcus by 1993 (Gardner and Schaffner, 1994). Health care providers are in the position to help prevent pneumococcal-related deaths by encouraging older people and family members to participate in the immunization program.

There are many pharmacological agents available that are used to treat pneumonia. There are standard guidelines for treating older persons with pneumonia (Table 6-2).

TABLE 6-2   Treatment Guidelines for the Elderly Patient with Pneumonia

Infection	Major Causative Organisms	Empiric Therapy	Comments
Community-acquired pneumonia	*Pneumococcus, Haemophilus, influenzae, Staphylococcus aureus* (also viruses, *Chlamydia, Legionella, Mycoplasma*)	Broad-spectrum antimicrobials	Consider aspiration pneumonia
Hospital-acquired pneumonia	Anaerobes and gram-negative organisms more likely to be involved	Aminoglycoside plus aminopenicillin (or cephalosporin with antipseudomonal activity) plus additional agents (e.g., vancomycin) if *Staphylococcus* is suspected	Elevate head of bed to prevent aspiration; monitor hygiene of endotracheal tubes
LTCF (long-term care facility)-acquired pneumonia	Colonization with gram-negative organisms more likely	Aminoglycoside plus aminopenicillin or clindamycin (if aspiration is likely)	Consider aspiration pneumonia, inadequate oral hygiene, impaired sensory perception

Source: *Reproduced with permission from R. N. Butler, T. J. Cali, D. B. Louria, M. A. Parrott, et al. (1994). Rational use of broad-spectrum antibiotics in the elderly. Geriatrics, 49 (supplement), S1–16.*

Prevention of pneumonia, rather than treatment, may need to be a more focused endeavor in health care settings. The incidence of hospital-acquired, or nosocomial, pneumonia demonstrates either a failure to prevent cross-contamination with infecting organisms or the transmission of more virulent organisms that may be antibiotic resistant (Levitzky, Cairo, and Hall, 1990). Proper handwashing and attention to infection control guidelines cannot be overemphasized.

Respiratory therapy equipment has historically played a role in the development of nosocomial respiratory tract infections. Within 22 hours of endotracheal intubation, gram-negative organisms can usually be cultured by secretions obtained from the lower respiratory tract. The widespread use of nebulizers with production of aerosols provides an excellent medium to transport contaminating organisms. Stethoscopes, which are routinely and frequently used, can transmit micro-organisms. Pulse oximeters carried from room to room and oxygen analyzer T-pieces reused between patients may be potential sources of contamination. Patient-to-patient spread of infection has been well-documented following the use of a Wright respirometer on several patients without proper disinfection techniques (Levitzky, Cairo, and Hall, 1990). The use of disposable, one-way valves is one way of reducing the chance of cross-contamination between patients (McPherson, 1995).

Older patients admitted to hospitals have depressed immune systems by virtue of their age alone. Frequently, these patients have a suboptimal nutritional status. Their ability to fight off and survive gram-negative nosocomial pneumonia is marginal. Prevention of nosocomial pneumonia—rather than treatment of the disease—would allocate time and resources more effectively.

Treatment for aspiration pneumonia varies, depending on the precipitating cause and the severity of lung involvement. Antibiotics are helpful when there is laboratory confirmation of a bacterial infection. Unfortunately, obtaining sputum specimens from older patients is often difficult. Because most community-acquired aspiration pneumonia responds well to penicillin—unless there is an allergy—it is usually the choice for empiric therapy (Dantzker, MacIntyre, and Bakow, 1995).

Due to the inflammatory reactions associated with aspiration pneumonia, corticosteroids are often used in the management of the disease. Fortunately, the inflammatory process is usually clinically insignificant after the first 72 hours if there is no secondary bacterial infection (Des Jardins and Burton, 1995). The administration of steroids early in the course of the disease seems to increase the rate of improvement in chest X-ray and arterial blood gas results. However, no long-term benefits, such as fewer complications or a reduced mortality rate, have been noted (Dantzker, MacIntyre, and Bakow, 1995). Despite the extensive use of corticosteroids to manage and treat aspiration pneumonia, their value remains controversial.

ACCIDENTS AND TRAUMA

Trauma is the fifth-leading cause of death among persons age 65 and older (Keough, Letizia, and Baldonado, 1994). While accidents are still more prevalent among younger age groups, especially teenagers, they are still responsible for a substantial number of deaths among older adults.

MOTOR VEHICLE ACCIDENTS

Auto accidents, especially among men, begin an upswing after midlife. It is possible that some of these, especially single-car accidents, represent suicide attempts (Thorson, 1995). Mortality from equally injuring accidents would, of course, be higher among older than among younger victims. It has been suggested that mortality statistics associated with trauma in the aged have been underestimated, as is demonstrated in this example:

> An older man is involved in a traffic accident and suffers a broken leg. He is admitted to the hospital and treated. Because he has a limited support system at home, he is discharged from the hospital into a nursing home. At the nursing home he becomes depressed, refuses to eat, refuses therapy, and becomes weak. In this state his immune system falters and he develops pneumonia. He eventually dies, but the death certificate lists the cause as pneumonia, not a broken leg.

FALLS

Among patients age 65 and older, falls are the most frequent cause of trauma (Table 6-3). One-third of community-dwelling older adults and a higher proportion of institutionalized elderly fall at least once annually.

Osteoporosis, or loss of bone mass, may lead to brittle bones in old age. Older people are less likely to have good balance. Their extremities are less padded by subcutaneous fat. Diminished sensory acuity (poor vision and hearing), dizziness, possible drug side effects, stroke, muscle weakness, and orthostatic hypotension can all lead to an increased likelihood of falls. Older people fall more often and their falls are more likely to result in hospitalization. The fractures leading to hospitalization most often are those of the upper femur

TABLE 6-3 Champion's Comparison of Age-Related Trauma Frequency/Mortality

	Patients Under Age 65		Patients Age 65 and Older	
	% Frequency	% Mortality	% Frequency	% Mortality
Falls	11	6	40.6	11.7
Motor vehicle accident	33.35	9.6	28.2	20.7
Pedestrian	7.9	13.5	10	32.6
Stab	11.9	4.7	2.6	17.3
Gun-shot wound	13	19.5	5.5	52.1
Motorcycle	7.7	11.9	0.4	11.8

Source: *Champion, 1989, as cited in Vicki Keough, Marijo Letizia, and Ardelina Baldonado, Facing the challenge of elderly trauma.* Journal of Gerontological Nursing, 20, *5–9. Reprinted by permission.*

and hip (Thorson, 1995). Bones of older people take longer to heal, often resulting in immobility, which can lead to **venostasis,** an impeded flow of blood in the veins, which can increase the risk of deep vein thrombosis and pulmonary embolism. Pulmonary embolism is an especially serious diagnosis in the elderly trauma victim (Keough, Letizia, and Baldonado, 1994).

Among all of the causes of trauma, except for motorcycle accidents, the percent mortality in the over 65 age group far exceeds the mortality rate for the same event for those younger than 65. Regardless of the type of trauma, this higher mortality rate is often associated with, and the result of, posttraumatic complications.

TRAUMA-ASSOCIATED COMPLICATIONS

Trauma-associated complications include emboli, sepsis, and pneumonia.

Pulmonary Embolism.   During the recuperative phase following trauma, immobility can eventually precipitate the formation of a **thrombus,** or blood clot. It is possible for this thrombus to form at the site of the trauma, and then loosen and travel through a vein to the lungs. The obstruction of any pulmonary vessel by a blood clot can lead to pulmonary embolism, an acute, life-threatening situation.

Sepsis.   Sepsis is one of the most serious complications associated with trauma. If the skin has been broken in any way, the barrier to infection has been compromised and bacteria may invade the body. The elderly have an increased susceptibility to certain viral and bacterial organisms because of changes in the immune system. One widely accepted theory is that older people have a delayed or inadequate response to infectious agents, so infections in the very old are more likely to be fatal than they are in younger persons (Hogstel, 1994a). This diminished immune response, which predisposes elderly patients to infection and sepsis, may also lead to multisystem organ failure.

Pneumonia.   Pneumonia is another complication of trauma among the elderly. In the majority of cases, it is associated with conditions in which there is significant impairment of the lungs' defense mechanisms (Farzan, 1992). Normal mucociliary clearance is slower in older patients. The cough reflex may also be weakened or ineffective, not just a result of old age but also as a consequence of trauma-associated immobility, pain, sedation, and dressings or binders. There is an alteration in the inflammatory response of older patients that results in an inadequate response to the stress of an infection. When sepsis is present, early signs and symptoms of a pneumonic process—such as a fever, pain, or an elevated white count—may not be present. By the time the patient is exhibiting obvious signs of distress, the pneumonia may be well advanced and difficult to treat. Diagnosis of pneumonia is generally more difficult with older patients, as the condition presents differently than it does among younger persons.

Adult Respiratory Distress Syndrome.   An acute form of respiratory failure, ARDS is characterized by diffuse damage at the alveolar level and altered permeability of the alveolar–capillary membrane. This condition may lead to inflammation, infiltration, edema, atelectasis, and alveolar hemorrhage. Pulmonary ARDS implies that the initial insult is to the lungs. Nonpulmonary causes of ARDS may be systemic, such as pancreatitis, uremia, or congestive heart failure. These and other conditions can ultimately lead to pulmonary involvement and/or failure.

Patients presenting with or developing rapidly progressive dyspnea, tachypnea, refractory hypoxemia, reduced lung volume, reduced compliance, or diffuse pulmonary infiltrates may have ARDS. Shock, burns, falls, accidents, sepsis, and aspiration are precipitating factors that could lead to ARDS in older persons. Fat embolism is another potential cause of ARDS. The majority of clinically recognizable cases of fat embolism follow multiple fractures, especially fractures of the long bones and pelvis (Farzan, 1992). The fat particles migrate from the bone marrow at the site of the fracture and enter the bloodstream at the site of the trauma through broken blood vessels. This process is enhanced if a manipulation of the fracture, in an attempt to reset it, is done. The fat particles (emboli) in the bloodstream become lodged in the tiny pulmonary vessels. The embolized fat undergoes hydrolysis and generates fatty acids. It is mainly the local chemical effect of fatty acids that causes diffuse pulmonary injury and an alteration in the alveolar–capillary membrane, resulting in ARDS. The incidence of falls in older adults and the disproportionate number of long-bone and pelvic fractures put the elderly in a higher risk group for fat emboli and resultant ARDS. ARDS is often fatal for older trauma patients.

Intervention.   Events that are unpredicted and unforeseen cannot always be prevented. Circumstances that might lead one to anticipate an accident, however, can be addressed. Prevention may take the form of education. Reinforcing safety measures with older people is often helpful. Preventive precautions such as avoiding abrupt motion (standing up slowly) and avoiding the use of high beds, throw rugs, and chairs with casters may help. Older people often have a hard time adapting to changes in light, particularly when going from the bright sunshine into a darker place. Taking time for the eyes to adjust may prevent a fall, as will well-lit stairs.

Older adults often have multiple chronic problems in addition to their acute situation. The older patient population presents a multifaceted challenge in the emergency setting and for the health care professional. An awareness of the posttraumatic complications common to this special population may change the course of treatment, facilitate generation of a comprehensive care plan, and hopefully result in a reduced mortality rate.

HYPOTHERMIA

An abnormally low body temperature is known as **hypothermia.** The most common cause of hypothermia is prolonged exposure to a cold environment. Normally, when the body temperature is low, the **hypothalamus** initiates a shivering response that generates heat. Unfortunately, the hypothalamus, the body's thermostat, does not always operate effectively among older adults (Thorson, 1995). If the shivering mechanism is not effective, not as much body heat will be generated. There is also a reduction in vasoconstriction in the elderly. The age-related loss of subcutaneous fat and the reduction of water in the tissues diminish normal insulating mechanisms. These factors all place the aged in a higher-risk group for complications associated with temperature extremes. Older people who are not able to keep their houses or apartments above 65°F may be prone to hypothermia. Especially at risk are the homeless elderly. There has been a great deal of attention focused on the problem of homelessness in the United States, but most of it is centered on the young homeless. A report based on eight cities across the United States estimated that 27 percent of the homeless are in fact over age 60 (Barrow, 1989). When an older person is suspected of having prolonged exposure to the cold, immediate treatment is imperative.

SIGNS AND SYMPTOMS

Recognizing clinical signs and symptoms of hypothermia early on may initiate appropriate intervention and increase the chances of survival. Because hypothermia reduces oxygen consumption and carbon dioxide production, persons with hypothermia may exhibit slow, shallow breathing and have reduced pulse rates (Scanlan, Spearman, and Sheldon, 1995). In addition to a low core body temperature (<93°F), other signs of hypothermia may include uncharacteristic confusion or drowsiness, a slow or irregular heartbeat, low blood pressure, and a lack of coordination.

Once a provisional diagnosis is made, rewarming is necessary. Gradual rewarming is recommended by warming the central (torso) part of the body before warming the extremities. Cardiac problems have been associated with rapidly sending cold blood back to the heart. Warm blankets and towels are very beneficial. In a hospital setting, warmed intravenous fluids are often prescribed. Delivery of warm, humidified gases can be used to treat hypothermia (Scanlan, Spearman, and Sheldon, 1995). Patients need to be monitored while being rewarmed. Temperature, pulse, respirations, and blood pressure should be checked frequently.

Recovery is dependent on a variety of conditions. Early intervention, the length of time the person was exposed to the cold, the core temperature when treatment was initiated, the status of health prior to the cold exposure, and the person's age are all significant factors. The average death rate from hypothermia for people 65 to 74 is almost four times the national average for all age groups. Those at greatest risk, adults age 85 and over, have a death rate nearly eight times higher than the national average (Hogstel, 1994b).

INTERVENTION

Given the independence of many older people, prevention of hypothermia is not always possible. Suggestions for avoiding hypothermia, such as using blankets and quilts when the thermostat cannot be turned up, wearing a loose-fitting cap or hat, and keeping legs and feet well covered, may or may not be heeded. Checking on elderly neighbors or relatives who live alone, especially during the coldest part of the year, can be lifesaving. It has been estimated that about 10 percent of the older people found dead at home during the winter months may have died of hypothermia (Thorson, 1995).

POSTOPERATIVE COMPLICATIONS

Numbers of older surgical patients are increasing in proportion to the growing geriatric population. Health care providers responsible for postoperative patient care need to be prepared for the increased numbers of geriatric surgical patients.

Coronary artery surgery is being performed increasingly in older and more seriously ill adults (Weintraub et al., 1991). Fortunately, there is an increased awareness of the risks and complications associated with surgery among older people. The elderly patient undergoing major cardiac surgery is unique in many ways. Fifty-five percent of the elderly have at least one or more other medical conditions in addition to their heart disease (Kern, 1991). Patients with coexisting renal insufficiency, diabetes, congestive heart failure, COPD, obesity, and a history of smoking are at increased risk when having heart surgery. Although cardiac surgery is one of the more common procedures, any surgical procedure in an older person adds an increased risk factor for morbidity and mortality. Diminished immunity and a blunted response to stress place the elderly in a higher risk category for complications. Even immobility prior to surgery can prolong the rate of recovery.

HYPERTENSION AND HYPOTHERMIA

During the immediate postoperative period, hypertension and hypothermia are major contributing factors that can lead to other complications (Whitman, 1991). Postoperative paroxysmal hypertension may present with a rapid onset immediately after surgery and can last up to 18 hours.

Endotracheal suctioning, pain, intolerance of the endotracheal tube or mechanical ventilator, arousal from anesthesia, hypoxia, and hypercapnia can exacerbate hypertension. Pharmacologic intervention is the most frequently used and most effective therapy for managing this type of hypertension. From a respiratory care standpoint, even though endotracheal suctioning is necessary, keeping the patient as comfortable as possible and assuring adequate ventilation may prevent the hypoxic/hypercapnic triggers that may play a role in ventilator intolerance.

Postoperative hypothermia is often a residual effect of intraoperative-induced hypothermia used to reduce the patient's oxygen requirements. It is another contributing factor in postsurgical complications. Older adults do not regulate their body temperatures as effectively as younger individuals. Not only is there a reduced **febrile** response in the aged but there is a diminished capacity to increase body temperature. One documented complication associated with induced hypothermia is hypothermic phrenic nerve injury. This transient effect on the phrenic nerve results in abnormal diaphragmatic movement and ultimately longer mechanical ventilation times and longer hospital stays (Dantzker, MacIntrye, and Bakow, 1995).

Consequences that may result during the rewarming maneuvers include overshoot hyperthermia, rewarming shock, and respiratory alterations (Whitman, 1991). Overshoot hyperthermia can result in tachycardia and increased oxygen consumption. Rewarming shock can result in severe hypotensive episodes. From a respiratory perspective, the most common problem in initially rewarming the patient is respiratory acidosis, which is due to low carbon dioxide production. As cardon dioxide production increases with rewarming, respiratory acidosis may become a problem. Slow, gradual rewarming of elderly patients and close attention to body temperatures to prevent overshoot hyperthermia is extremely important. Ventilator management of postoperative patients may need to include manipulation of the minute ventilation to ward off problems associated with rewarming-induced respiratory acidosis.

RESPIRATORY COMPLICATIONS

Respiratory complications are the primary cause of morbidity after major surgical procedures and a leading cause of death in older patients (Scanlan, Spearman, and Sheldon, 1995). Maintaining a patent airway, with or without an adjunct artificial airway, is a high priority in all postsurgical patients.

Preventing hypoxemia may avoid an entire cascade of adverse events. Older patients have a low tolerance for even small airway obstructions, which is due in part to loss of tone of the respiratory muscles, but also to a decreased surface area for gas exchange, which has already reduced their ability to oxygenate blood. Decreased cardiac outputs and anemia as a result of postsurgical blood volume depletion or even a preexisting condition will increase the older patient's vulnerability to hypoxemia. Oxygen saturation and arterial blood partial pressure monitoring, along with the delivery of enough oxygen to assure adequate tissue oxygenation, is imperative.

Postoperative Atelectasis.   Postoperative atelectasis is another way that tissue oxygenation may be compromised. Atelectasis is the most common postoperative pulmonary complication. It affects about a quarter of all patients recovering from abdominal or thoracic surgery. Atelectasis, a failure of part of the lungs to expand, usually develops during the first or second postoperative day. Contributing factors in the aged are shallow breathing, obstruction of the airway with secretions, pain (which results in smaller tidal volumes), immobility, a transient decrease in surfactant production, a weakened cough reflex, and decreased ciliary movement (Scanlan, Spearman, and Sheldon, 1995). Atelectasis as a result of any of these factors can lead to a mismatching of ventilation and perfusion, and thus to arterial hypoxemia.

Areas of alveolar collapse, or atelectasis, are prone to infection. If an area of the lung remains atelectatic for greater than 72 hours, pneumonia is likely to develop. In the elderly, aggressive prophylactic measures to prevent atelectasis are preferable to treating the pneumonia that may result from it.

Frequent incentive spirometry maneuvers with an inspiratory hold, turning every 2 hours, and early ambulation—as soon as the vital signs are stable—are important therapeutic interventions (Figure 6-2). Pain management without the use of sedatives that depress respirations will also help to prevent alveolar compromise.

If atelectasis does develop, strategies such as administration of chest physiotherapy and postural drainage for secretion removal, hyperinflation therapy such as IPPB (intermittent positive pressure breathing) or CPAP (continuous positive airway pressure), and even

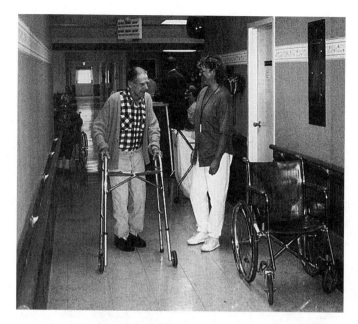

Figure 6-2 *Ambulation in older adults can often be therapeutic.*

moderate nasotracheal suctioning may help reverse atelectasis and aid in reexpansion of the lungs (Figure 6-3).

Aspiration Pneumonia.   Aspiration pneumonia is a very serious postsurgical problem. Two-thirds of all aspiration events follow thoracic or abdominal surgery (Scanlan, Spearman, and Sheldon, 1995). Dysphagia postoperatively is a serious and often unrecognized problem. Aspiration of food and fluid can occur in the aged, the intubated, and the patient with diminished consciousness. It is estimated that up to 12 percent of hospitalized patients have dysphagia and that 70 percent of all people with diminished consciousness microaspirate (Kern, 1991). It has also been estimated that about 50 percent of aspiration events result in pneumonia and that over 30 percent of patients with gross aspiration progressing to pneumonia die as a result of it, although it is a totally preventable complication.

Postoperative Infections.   Postoperative infections are another complicating factor that can increase patient morbidity and mortality. Bacterial contamination of the sternum is the most common infectious problem associated with cardiac surgery. It appears to be age related. Studies indicate that sternal infections increase in direct proportion to the age of the patient (Weintraub et al., 1991; Vaca, Lohmann, and Moskoff, 1994).

Sepsis in the intensive care unit in elderly postsurgical and posttraumatic patients is also a problem for all of the reasons that have been mentioned. Protocols for preventing the infections that lead to sepsis go back to the basics: handwashing.

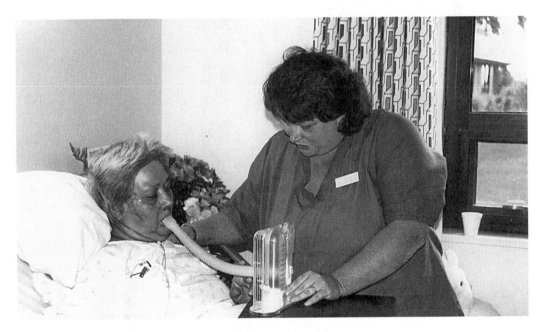

Figure 6-3 *Hyperinflation therapy on a postsurgical older patient.*

Some additional strategies in critical care settings include isolation procedures, antibiotic use when necessary, adequate nutritional support, and strict adherence to sterile suctioning techniques. Respiratory therapists who routinely suction post-CABG (coronary art bypass graft) patients should cover the sternal wound with a plastic barrier (Chux) to protect and keep the wound dry whenever ventilator tubing is disconnected from the endotracheal tube. Moisture seeping onto the gauze dressing will reduce the barrier to bacterial contamination and increase the incidence of sepsis (Kern, 1991).

SUMMARY

Respiratory care of the acutely ill elderly patient incorporates many procedures and involves many principles of management. Regardless of the diagnosis and prescribed treatment, in geriatric medicine the procedures must be tailored to fit the patient. Age-related physiological changes must be considered. Altered sensoriums must be evaluated and dealt with realistically and compassionately. New technology and research continually add to the arsenal of medical advances we have at our disposal. Expanding the knowledge base of health care providers to include geriatric care is an imperative. Although advanced age is clearly a factor in mortality, preparedness may reduce the complications that lead to mortality. Education and preparation are the logical approaches to improving the quality of acute care for older adults.

Review Questions

1. What acute diseases are associated with a higher mortality rate in the elderly population?
2. Compare and contrast symptoms of an AMI in a 40-year-old female and an 80-year-old female.
3. Outline the management options in an elderly patient who presents with an AMI.
4. Diagnostically, what will help distinguish between an acute exacerbation of asthma, emphysema, and chronic bronchitis in an older adult?
5. Why is the mortality rate higher in older adults who suffer from a traumatic event such as an accident?
6. It is 2:10 A.M. An 80-year-old homeless man has just been brought into the emergency room complaining of shortness of breath. His SpO_2 on room air is 85 percent. His body temperature is 94°F. Describe your actions in detail on how you would proceed to help this patient.
7. What possible complication should you be on guard against in an 85-year-old post-surgical patient?

References

Barnett, L., Harnett, P. T., and Bond, A. F. (1992). Patterns of emergency department use by geriatric patients. *Journal of Gerontological Social Work, 19,* 77–96.

Barrow, G. (1989). *Aging, the individual, and society.* St. Paul, MN: West.

Bills, G., and Soderberg, R. (1994). *Principles of pharmacology for respiratory care.* Albany, NY: Delmar.

Bloom, H. G., and Shlom, E. A. (1993). *Drug prescribing for the elderly.* New York: Raven Press.

Brown, K. K. (1995). Surgical therapy of chronic heart failure and severe ventricular dysfunction. *Critical Care Nursing Quarterly, 18,* 45–55.

Butler, R. N. (1994). Pneumococcal vaccine is worth a shot. *Geriatrics, 49,* 9–11.

Chesi, G., Pinelli, G., Galimberti, O., Navazio, A., and Montanari, P. (1994). Effectiveness of nasal positive pressure ventilation in the management of acute refractory left ventricular insufficiency. *Minerva-Cardioangiol, 42* (4), 149–155.

Dantzker, D. R., MacIntyre, N. R., and Bakow, E. D. (1995). *Comprehensive respiratory care.* Philadelphia: W. B. Saunders.

deLarminat, V., Montravers, P., Dureuil, B., and Desmonts, J-M. (1995). Alteration in swallowing reflex after extubation in intensive care unit patients. *Critical Care Medicine, 23,* 486–490.

Des Jardins, T., and Burton, G. G. (1995). *Clinical manifestations and assessment of respiratory disease.* St. Louis, MO: Mosby.

Eubanks, D. H., and Bone, R. C. (1990). *Comprehensive respiratory care.* St. Louis, MO: Mosby.

Farzan, S. (1992). *A concise handbook of respiratory diseases.* Norwalk, CT: Appleton and Lange.

Fulmer, T. T., and Walker, M. K. (1990). Lessons from the elder boom in ICU. *Geriatric Nursing, 11,* 120.

Gardner, P., and Schaffner, W. (1994). Immunization of adults. *New England Journal of Medicine, 328,* 1252–1258.

Hazzard, W. R., Bierman, E. L., Glass, J. P., Eltinger, W. H., and Halter, J. B. (1994). *Principles of geriatric medicine and gerontology,* 3rd ed. New York: McGraw-Hill.

Hellman, E. A., and Williams, M. A. (1994). Outpatient cardiac rehabilitation in elderly patients. *Heart and Lung, 23,* 506–511.

Hogstel, M. O. (1994a). *Nursing care of the older adult.* Albany, NY: Delmar.

Hogstel, M. O. (1994b). Vital signs are really vital in the old-old. *Geriatric Nursing, 15* (5), 252–255.

Keough, V., Letizia, M., and Baldonado, A. (1994). *Journal of Gerontological Nursing, 20,* 5–11.

Kern, L. S. (1991). The elderly heart surgery patient. *Critical Care Nursing Clinics of North America, 3,* 749–756.

Kyes, K. (1994). Geriatric asthma—A conversation with Benjamin Burrows, MD. *RT—The Journal for Respiratory Care Practitioners, 7* (3), 31–38.

Lamy, P. P. (1980). *Prescribing for the elderly.* Littleton, MA: PSG Publishing.

Levitzky, M. G., Cairo, J. M., and Hall, S. M. (1990). *Introduction to respiratory care.* Philadelphia: W. B. Saunders.

Louria, D. B. (1994). Roundtable discussion: Rational use of broad-spectrum antibiotics in the elderly. *Geriatrics, 49* (supplement), S1–14.

Marieb, E. N. (1992). *Human anatomy and physiology.* Redwood City, CA: Benjamin/Cummings.

McPherson, S. P. (1995). *Respiratory care equipment.* St. Louis, MO: Mosby.

Miziniak, H. (1994). Persons with Alzheimer's: Effects of nutrition and exercise. *Journal of Gerontological Nursing, 20* (10), 27–29.

Needham, J. F. (1993). *Gerontological nursing: A restorative approach.* Albany, NY: Delmar.

O'Brien-Ladner, A. (1994). Asthma: New insights in the management of older adults. *Geriatrics, 49,* 20–32.

Odeh, M., Oliven, A., and Bassan, H. (1991). Timolol eyedrop-induced fatal bronchospasm in an asthmatic patient. *The Journal of Family Practice 32,* 97–98.

Pearl, J. (1994). Roundtable discussion: Rational use of broad-spectrum antibiotics in the elderly. *Geriatrics, 49* (supplement), S1–14.

Raiha, I. J., Ivaska, K., and Sourander, L. B. (1992). Pulmonary function in gastro-esophageal reflux disease of elderly people. *Age and Ageing, 21,* 368–373.

Scanlan, C. L., Spearman, C., and Sheldon, R. L. (1995). *Fundamentals of respiratory care.* St. Louis, MO: Mosby.

Sobol, E., and Fleming, R. (1994, Dec.). Treating the aged. *Advance for Managers of Respiratory Care, 3* (12), 41–43.

Spence, A. P. (1989). *Biology of human aging.* Englewood Cliffs, NJ: Prentice-Hall.

Thorson, J. A. (1995). *Aging in a changing society.* Belmont, CA: Wadsworth.

Tierney, L. M., McPhee, S. J., and Papadakis, M. A. (1995). *Current medical diagnosis and treatment.* Norwalk, CT: Appleton and Lange.

Tsuyuki, R. T., Ikuta, R. M., Greenwood, P. V., and Montague, T. J. (1994). Mortality risk and patterns of practice in 2,070 patients with acute myocardial infarction, 1987–92. *Chest, 105,* 1687–1692.

Vaca, K. J., Lohmann, D. P., and Moskoff, M. E. (1994). Cardiac surgery in the octogenarian: Nursing implications. *Heart Lung, 23,* 413–422.

Weintraub, W. S., Craver, J. M., Cohen, C. L., Jones, E. L., and Guyton, R. A. (1991). Influence of age on results of coronary artery surgery. *Circulation, 84,* 226–235.

Whitman, G. R. (1991). Hypertension and hypothermia in the acute postoperative period. *Critical Care Nursing Clinics of North America, 3,* 661–673.

CHAPTER SEVEN

LONG-TERM CARE

collaborative self-management
failure to thrive
hospice

institutionalization
social death

social worth
spend-down

— LEARNING OBJECTIVES —

After completing this chapter, the reader should be able to:

1. List some of the predictors of institutionalization among the elderly.
2. Recognize prevailing societal attitudes toward nursing homes.
3. Recognize the impact of perceived social worth on patient care.
4. Name some of the outcomes of transfer trauma.
5. Give signs of failure to thrive among older institutionalized patients.
6. Describe the predictors of elder abuse.

INTRODUCTION

Respiratory care in geriatrics often involves the care of people who will not recover from the particular illness or illnesses they have. Health problems may be with them for an extended period of time, perhaps for the rest of their lives. Long-term care usually implies institutionalization. However, long-term care could as easily take place in the home as within a subacute setting or a nursing home. Emphasizing in-home care is a trend in the field. The stated goal of many services for the elderly has been to maximize independence, to provide alternatives to institutionalization, and to keep people at home for as long as possible.

There are several good reasons for this goal, most of which revolve around the meaning behind the message associated with institutionalization.

NURSING HOMES

The growth of nursing homes—both in number of facilities and number of residents—has hit a plateau in the United States. After several decades of rapid growth, the rate of new development of nursing homes has declined for several reasons. One is that the cost of nursing home care has become very expensive. Few families will turn to nursing homes until they have exhausted other options. Second, there are other resources; home health care agencies and service programs for the elderly have grown in recent decades, and they have been successful at delaying nursing home entry. Third, state governments are required by federal regulation to limit the growth of health care facilities through the process of issuing certificates of need. An investigation and hearing is required before any new hospital or nursing home can be built. The reasoning is that third-party payers (insurance companies and government reimbursement plans such as Medicaid and Medicare) essentially foot the major part of the bill for construction of new facilities. It would be poor economics to continue to pay for new hospitals and nursing homes where there is no particular need for them.

The most recent National Health Provider Inventory (Sirrocco, 1994) distinguishes actual nursing homes from some 31,431 board and care homes, about half of which are for the mentally retarded. These typically are not true nursing homes. Board and care homes serve about half a million people in the United States.

There are 16,700 nursing homes in the United States (Strahan, 1997). They serve slightly over 1.5 million people per year. About 80 percent of these nursing homes have fifty or more beds. Two-thirds of them are proprietary (profit-making). Costs for nursing home care currently run from about $3,000 per month to over $4,500 in some major cities. Thus, one of the incentives for keeping a relative home as long as possible is financial, as few people have nursing home insurance and Medicare typically does not pay for most nursing home care.

The fear many people have is that their personal finances will be quickly exhausted by the high costs of nursing home care and that they will be forced to go on Medicaid, which is possible only after spending down their own resources. This **spend-down** actually happens in only about 20 percent of the cases (Liu and Manton, 1991), which indicates that families are often successful in keeping their older members out of nursing homes for as long as humanly possible (Brody, 1985).

There are some predictors of who will be placed in a nursing home. Those who live alone, obviously, are more likely. Age also predicts nursing home entry—the older, the more likely to be in a nursing home. Being female is a predictor of placement, as women are less likely to have a surviving spousal caregiver (Figure 7-1). Being cared for by family members other than a spouse is a predictor due to lower morale and higher perceived stress among family caregivers. Help for the family such as respite and home health care significantly extends the family's ability to care for their elder member at home and ultimately keep costs lower (Kosloski and Montgomery, 1995). The presence of Alzheimer's

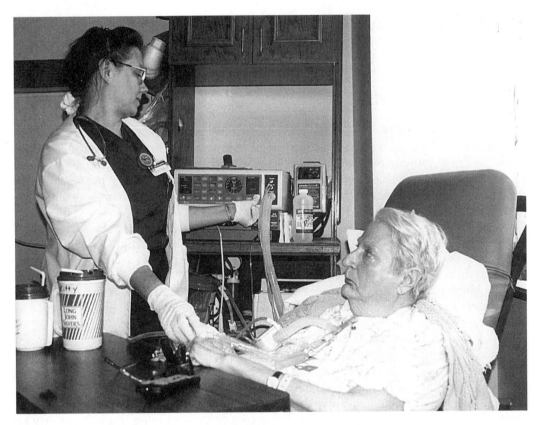

Figure 7-1 *Patients in long-term care are much more likely to be female.*

disease is also a predictor of nursing home entry (Montgomery and Kosloski, 1994). In fact, the majority of nursing home patients are there because of some form of dementia.

THE MESSAGE OF INSTITUTIONALIZATION

It may be difficult for younger people to visualize a distant future when they are very old and frail, when just getting to and from the bathroom is a struggle, when a host of aches and pains and medical problems dominates every waking moment. Suddenly, an acute problem—say, a stroke or a broken hip—means a trip to the hospital. After a fairly brief course of acute care, what happens? It might be impossible to go directly from the hospital to home. The next step for many people is from the hospital into a nursing home. For many, the inevitable message of admission to a nursing home is that it may be the last stop before death.

ATTITUDES TOWARD NURSING HOMES

There is the inevitable message associated with nursing homes of decline, failure, and dissolution. While the best facilities emphasize rehabilitation and many facilities provide sympathetic care for people in great need, there still is the social message that long-term care facilities represent a holding place for those who are about to die.

Despite the rehabilitation motive, the inevitability is that most nursing home patients do indeed die, usually within a relatively brief period of time after admission. This, of course, is because only the sickest of the sick reside in nursing homes. These are people who are nearing the end of their lives. No one can be rehabilitated forever, and even the best efforts at restoration must ultimately fail.

However, another prevailing attitude in society is that health care institutions are designed to cure people and return them to their homes. The cure motive is emphasized to such an extent that the important other motive of health care—the function of caring—is too often forgotten. A more realistic attitude would be to see places where people are taken care of until they die as beneficial. Most members of an aging population will eventually need such care.

Societal Trends.   The trend over the past decade is for patients to be discharged sicker and more frail from acute care hospitals because of prospective payment plans and diagnostic-related groups. For this reason, the kind of patients now seen in nursing homes is different from the typical patient mix even a few years ago. This situation means heavier nursing and more involvement of other allied health professionals. It also means that a higher proportion of nursing home patients will be there for terminal care. The nursing home is ultimately emerging as a hospice, whether this is intentional or not.

SOCIAL WORTH AND SOCIAL DEATH

An inevitable problem of care within institutions is a perceived impersonality or coldness, which goes beyond the physical coldness of tile floors and long corridors. A lack of interpersonal warmth is typical where multitudes of strangers troop in and out of patient rooms, often without identifying themselves or acknowledging the personhood of the very individual they mean to serve. This is particularly the case in hospitals, but it is true as well in other health care institutions.

The best people working in institutions are aware of this problem and strive to minimize it, but even the best institutions are still institutions. By their nature, institutions have to follow certain regimens and bureaucratic patterns to operate efficiently. These procedures, rules, and regulations often can be dehumanizing. Also, there are natural human tendencies that can exacerbate the problems inherent in institutional care.

One of the most disturbing of these tendencies is the unspoken assignment of **social worth** to patients. At its most basic level, this assignment of social value or social worth means that people who are seen as more important get better care and people at the bottom of the social ladder are more likely to be ignored. This concept was first identified by David Sudnow (1967) in his sociological studies of death in hospitals. Sudnow observed that emergency room medicine, for example, followed not only the triage concept of giving medical priority to those most in need of it, but that well-dressed people tended to receive quicker and better care than did those perceived as lower on the social scale, say, drug addicts or derelicts.

A present-day example of high social worth at work in a health care setting would be former New York Yankee baseball player Mickey Mantle receiving a transplantable liver after a wait of just 2 days in the summer of 1995. He received a second liver transplant when the first one failed, but he died a month later. Officials at Baylor University Medical Center took pains to claim that it was not Mantle's fame and high status that moved him up the transplant list. This was laughable to most observers—and no doubt bitter news to those who had been waiting many months for a liver. One would only need to compare how quickly a 63-year-old alcoholic who was *not* famous would have to wait for an organ transplant to see the importance of social worth in action.

In Sudnow's (1967) research, there were many signs of high social worth other than fame or prosperity. People in the hospital who had many visitors tended to be seen as higher in social value than those who had none. Those who were lucid and who could communicate tended to be better cared for on an interpersonal level than those who were comatose or demented. Younger and better-looking people were preferred over the aged or the disfigured. Patients with higher social worth enjoyed quicker response to their call lights. Staff tended to talk more with them and spend more time with them. People who were expected to recover tended to have a higher status than those the staff expected to die. Thus, nearness to death was seen as an indicator of declining social value.

CASE STUDY

The staff at the nursing home often said that Ms. Katie Black looked very much like a turkey: She had a peaked nose that came down much like a beak and loose skin on her skinny old neck that flapped back and forth when she jerked her head around in a birdlike manner, which she did frequently. And she sort of gobbled. She sounded pretty strange. Because she could make no sense when she tried to speak, some of the care staff members had given up trying to communicate with her and found that they instead talked *about* her to each other, even while they were giving her physical care. Her behavior was seen as hopelessly bizarre and the care she received became increasingly mechanical.

One day while feeding her, it was apparent that she was trying to say something. One of us said to her, "Katie, I just can't understand you." And she replied in a perfectly clear, crisp voice, "I know. Isn't it terrible?" Then she started to gobble again. When told of Ms. Black's one moment of clear speech, her brief success at communication, the rest of the staff was amazed. Although she never again mastered the ability to speak, her care from that point on became more personalized, almost as if she had rejoined the world of the living.

The dying in Sudnow's observation were treated as being less important patients. Their doctors tended to lose interest in them when it became clear that a cure was not possible. They were seen by fewer and fewer people—both visitors and staff members—as they went along a trajectory toward death, finally interacting with perhaps one or two relatives and one or two caregivers. The rest of the world had disengaged from them. The sad message was that the ones nearest to death were in fact left alone to die.

This isolation is one of the factors that makes **institutionalization** distasteful to most people. It is the reason that most people, when given a choice, would prefer to live—and die—at home. Not only is the institutional environment foreign but interpersonal interaction is inevitably stilted in institutional settings. Institutions have their own norms and mores. Their procedures take away freedom.

CASE STUDY

Some years ago, one of the authors of this text worked in a nursing home. It was a good one; it provided good nursing care and had an enviable record of rehabilitation of its residents. Residents were sorted in terms of their physical location in the institution by their level of incapacity. This is not an uncommon practice for nursing homes or for hospitals. In this case, those who were the least sick had rooms at the end of the corridor that was closest to the main part of the building with the cafeteria, administrative offices, visiting room, and other places of coming and going. This made sense—those people were the likeliest to use those facilities. They were, for example, able to go on their own to the dining room for their meals.

The opposite end of the corridor housed the sickest and most serious residents. They all had to be fed, so it made sense that they did not need rooms closest to the dining room. They were in the patient rooms adjacent to the nurses' station. This also made sense—the heaviest nursing cases were more efficiently located nearest to where the nurses were. This logically would cut down on the time it took personnel to get to the rooms of these patients as well as the expenditure of staff energy.

Down at the very end of the wing were the people who were demented and who could not communicate. It became second nature in these cases for the staff members to not speak to these individuals when they entered the room. It is difficult to carry on a one-way conversation; when communication is not rewarded with a response, the tendency is to not communicate at all. A real indication of declining social worth, however, was when two or more staff members would enter one of these rooms, they not only would avoid speaking to the resident but they often would talk with each other *about* the resident. This took place in many different circumstances and the physicians often were the worst examples. It was common for them to talk to the nursing staff members about a patient in his or her presence without even acknowledging the individual.

Talking about people in their presence is a sure sign of the low social worth accorded to them. Taking this one step along an inevitable conceptual path, it could be said that people whose social worth becomes low enough could actually be said to be socially dead. **Social death** in an institution often occurs prior to actual physical death. Social death is when the individual is treated as an object rather than a person.

In the example of the nursing home, those patients nearest the nurses' station frequently were treated as socially dead. In this particular instance, there was an empty room at the very end of the corridor where dead bodies were wrapped. So, it was literally possible for a person to enter the nursing home at one end and then be moved progressively down the corridor toward the empty room as physical condition deteriorated. It was well known that those nearest the empty room were the ones expected to die soon, and the residents as well as the staff were aware of this.

RELOCATION AND TRANSFER TRAUMA

It has been known for some time that there is a dramatically elevated death rate among elderly people shortly after admission to nursing homes (Blenkner, 1967). A large proportion of those deaths takes place in a relatively short time after admission. Liu and Manton (1984) found that, among a 1-year nursing home entry cohort nationally of 1.1 million persons, 24 percent had died within the first 30 days after admission, and an additional 30 percent of those remaining died within the next 60 days.

The stereotype of older people living in nursing homes for years and years is just that— a stereotype. It is perpetuated because the relatively small group that does live on for years in institutional settings are those who are visible. They represent the minority, however. There actually are three groups of patients in long-term-care institutions: those who remain there for an extended period of time, those who are rehabilitated and return home, and those who die there. Some facilities have an enviable record of restoring frail and disabled older persons to independence by utilizing extensive rehabilitation services. On the other hand, there are also long-term-care facilities that have no rehabilitation services at all and have only two kinds of patients: those who die sooner and those who die later.

It should be recognized that tracking the history of nursing home patients is a very difficult thing to do. It has been common practice in many long-term-care institutions for patients to be sent to the hospital when they become seriously ill or near the point of death. It is then an economic necessity for most facilities to fill that empty bed as soon as possible— not to hold it for the patient who may or may not return. As a result, many people who are institutionalized may have multiple relocations during their final year of life—from nursing home to hospital, from hospital to another nursing home, perhaps back to the same or to another hospital, home for a brief period of time, and then back to another institution, and so on.

Lewis and her colleagues (1985) recognized this problem. They followed a random sample of 197 persons from 24 different nursing homes for 2 years. Only 9 percent of the patients were discharged to their homes and received no further institutional care during that period of time. A total of 37 percent died in the nursing home to which they had first been admitted, and 54 percent were transferred frequently between hospitals and other nursing homes. Over 72 percent of the original group had died by the end of the 2-year period, and only 15 percent were alive and living at home at the end of 2 years. The remaining 13 percent were living in a skilled care setting. Only 28 percent were still alive at the end of the study period. There was a death rate of over 72 percent within 2 years of nursing home admission.

One cannot, though, conclude from these data that the stress associated with admission to a nursing home might have precipitated death among those who could otherwise have lived on for some time. There is no way to know if these patients might have died if they had remained at home. This research problem was first described by Margaret Blenkner

(1967), who speculated that the environmental change associated with institutionalization was the causal factor for the high mortality rate. She reviewed studies of populations of the frail elderly who had been moved from one institution to another in an attempt to hold constant the effects of institutionalization so as to study the effect of relocation itself. Her review led her to the conclusion that there was a significant effect from relocation, particularly among those with what at that time was called chronic brain syndrome.

The conclusion from Blenkner's research was that the focus of services to older people should be to keep them out of institutions for as long as possible, to provide them with services that maximize independence, and to provide alternatives to institutionalization. Since that time there have been numerous studies confirming the negative effects of involuntary transfer. "It appears that the degree of environmental change involved in relocation is an important factor influencing the mortality rate. Anticipation of relocation may be nearly as lethal as the relocation itself" (Bourestom and Tars, 1974). This situation could be due to the perception of the threat of loss of personal control. It could be that the stress of an anticipated move, and having no say in it, precipitates death among an already frail group. This would be consistent with the findings of other researchers.

Locus of control was discussed in Chapter 2. Loss of personal decision-making power might be perceived by some people as overwhelmingly stressful. Taking personal control away from people might be seen as a way of reinforcing their low social worth. Deciding things for people implies that they are no longer capable of making decisions for themselves. The situation of a nursing home patient whose daughter sold his car—and then told him about it later—is illustrative. The message he perceived was that she was in charge now, his opinion did not matter, and he would never emerge from the nursing home again to be driving that car. The old man died shortly thereafter. "The sense of control, the illusion that one can exercise personal choice, has a definite and positive role in sustaining life" (Lefcourt, 1973, p. 424).

Failure to Thrive.   Older people who have lost a sense of personal control may lose the will to live. An important contribution to the gerontological literature was made by three nurse researchers (Braun, Wykle, and Cowling, 1988), who pointed out that this effect is similar to the **failure to thrive** syndrome seen among institutionalized children.

At one time in our history, about two generations ago, large orphanages were a typical part of the scene in every city. They are no longer there. It was discovered that children raised in orphanages had a higher death rate, lower average intelligence, and did not do as well physically or emotionally as children who lived in families. The standard approach with children who have no suitable home environment now is to find them another one, either through adoption or through foster care.

Braun and her colleagues state that,

The term *failure to thrive* first appeared in the pediatric literature in reference to institutionalized infants who slowly and then rapidly lost weight (Holt, 1897). Early descriptions of failing infants included the symptom complex "listlessness, relative immobility, quietness, indifferent appetite, failure to gain weight, and the appearance of unhappiness" (Bakwin, 1949). In turn, failure to thrive among elderly persons may, perhaps, mirror the pediatric phenomenon. It is not uncommon to find nursing home residents who gradually lose weight, decline in physical and cognitive function, withdraw from social activity, and exhibit an indifferent appetite. Frequently, staff are stymied in their attempts to encourage adequate nutritional intake and to arrest or reverse the decline. (1988, p. 809)

The authors go on to cite parallels between younger and older institutionalized persons, and they use the term "giving up" to describe both groups. They state that the combination of helplessness and hopelessness leads to higher rates of infection in both younger and older institutionalized populations. They point to the concept of "psychogenic mortality" among the aged, a syndrome where a person's psychological condition triggers physical effects "of a pathogenic nature leading ultimately to death," a phenomenon remarkably like the giving-up complex seen in children with failure to thrive (1988, p. 811). They also note that the effectiveness of many different attempted interventions has yet to be shown. Touch seems to be important, but oftentimes the institutionalized older person is of such low social value as to be starved for touch (Figure 7-2).

Maizler, Solomon, and Almquist (1983) recommend intensive nursing intervention. Persons who feel isolated quite logically need to receive the message that they are *not* isolated.

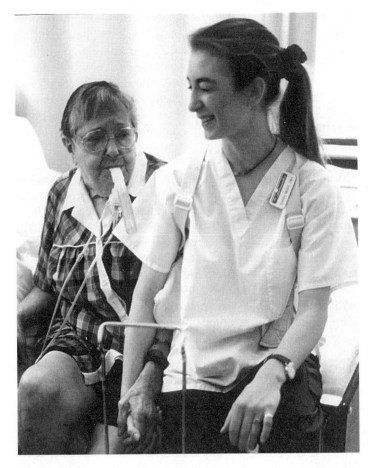

Figure 7-2 *Older people need touch.*

Unfortunately, the staffing patterns in most nursing homes are such that intensive nursing intervention is not a realistic possibility.

In one of the early articles on alienation and the loss of the will to live, Ellison (1969) suggested that the root cause is social isolation. Institutionalization by itself does not impose isolation, but it certainly exacerbates it. About 20 percent of the aged have no children (7 percent of the elderly never married and 13 percent married but were childless). However, roughly 40 percent of the elderly who are in nursing homes are childless. This statistic implies that those who are childless are about twice as likely to wind up in a nursing home. Anxiety and loneliness are some of the common emotional states that health care professionals look for during patient assessment (Figure 7-3).

Implications.   One implication is that successful intervention with nursing home residents might include an assessment of how socially engaged or isolated they are (Figure 7-4). Do they have family members? Do the family members visit? Do they have other social contacts, or are they alone? Then a special effort must be made by all members of the interdisciplinary health care team to spend more time with those who are at greatest risk of social isolation. Time must be taken to sit down and talk, touch, and develop a relationship. Bringing small gifts, something even as minor as a newspaper, can be an effective way of entering an individual's social world. Institutionalized people who are isolated from the outside community and ignored by staff and other patients have the highest risk of losing the will to live.

HOSPICE

The first modern institution devoted to specialized care of the terminally ill, St. Christopher's in London, was named a **hospice** because religious orders established hospices in the Middle Ages along pilgrim routes. They were places for people who were on a journey, and often sick pilgrims would find the hospice to be the end of their personal journey. Many of the institutions developed in the last century—poor farms, tuberculosis sanitariums, asylums—really were places in which to isolate the ill. However, it is only within the past generation or so that institutional support for the terminally ill has emerged.

The hospice is not only intentional about caring for dying people, it has a special goal of seeing that they are not isolated at the end of their lives. The first American hospice was founded in 1972 in New Haven, Connecticut. Since that time, about 2,000 different hospice programs have been developed in various places in the United States. A hospice does not necessarily have to have a building—home health and visiting nurse programs deliver most hospice care. However, hospice is often thought of as a place as well as a program. Nursing homes can have a designated section that is called a hospice, as can hospitals. For federal reimbursement, the most desirable thing is to have acute care (hospital care), chronic care (nursing home), and home health care under one organizational umbrella. This is an ideal but not a practical impediment to organizational development. Many hospice programs reimbursed by Medicare are simply patched together from two or three different organizations.

CAT.	ACTIVATION		ACTUAL	POTEN.	NO	PROBLEM	RESOLUTION		REACTIVATION		RESOLUTION	
	DATE	INI-TIALS					DATE	INI-TIALS	DATE	INI-TIALS	DATE	INI-TIALS
S E N S O R Y					1.	Cognitive Alteration						
					2.	Communication Alteration						
					3.	Confusion/Disorientation						
					4.	Sensory Alteration						
G E N E R A L					5.	BODY FLUIDS:						
					6.	NUTRITION:						
					7.	BOWEL:						
					8.	BLADDER:						
S K I N					9.	SKIN:						
					10.	Infection/Inflammation						
S Y M P T O M C O N T.					11.	Discomfort/Pain						
					12.	Rest/Sleep						
					13.	Medication Tolerance						
					14.	RESPIRATORY:						
					15.	CARDIAC:						
F U N C. L I M.					16.	Weakness Endurance Vertigo						
					17.	MOBILITY:						
					18.	SELF-CARE ACTIVITIES: Alteration in Ability To Perform ADL's/Personal Care						
					19.	Comatose						
P S Y C H O L O G I C A L					20.	Anger						
					21.	Anxiety/Fear/Depression/Irritability						
					22.	Alterations in Body Language						
					23.	Loneliness/Isolation						
					24.	Grieving/Bereavement						
					25.	Spiritual Concerns						
					26.	Client/Family/Caretaker Problems						
					27.	Coping of Client/Family/Caretaker						
					28.	Noncompliance with Care Plan						
					29.	Lack of Knowledge Re:						
					30.	Economic/Financing Options						
					31.	Will/Funeral Arrangements						
O T H E R					32.							
					33.							
					34.							
					35.							
					36.							
					37.							
					38.							
					39.							
					40.							
					41.							
					42.							
					43.							

Imprint Client Identification or Write-In Information Below

PROBLEM LIST
Refer to Reverse Side for Signature List

Client's Name

Client Record No.

Home Care Project/FORE of AMRA 5/86 Form #8

Figure 7-3 *Model form for recording patient problems. (Source: Amy Marie Haddad (1987).* High tech home care. *Rockville, MD: Aspen. Reprinted with permission.)*

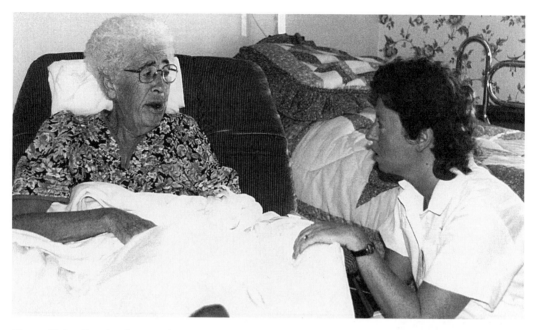

Figure 7-4 *Emotional status should be included in patient assessment.*

The goal of hospice is to provide compassionate care to the dying (Figure 7-5). Entering hospice care essentially is entering an open awareness. Denial of impending death no longer gets in the way of effective communication. People are no longer pretending that the individual will recover, so they can get past the common platitudes and actually talk about what is important. What people often find to be most important—a concept that is developed more fully in Chapter 8—is unfinished business. It may be the health care professional's job—although this will never appear in a job description—to help dying people accomplish their unfinished business.

It may also be the health care professional's job to sit down and listen when an individual wants to share some personal history. Listening can be effective therapy. Never let the mechanics of the job dominate or take precedence over interpersonal contact. The therapist's job is to provide therapy, whether it involves administering oxygen or sitting down and listening to some person's thoughts on the value of his or her life. Too often, health care professionals project an image of being too busy to take the time for what is really important, when giving someone just an extra minute or two would develop genuine human contact.

Again, this contact is one of the goals of hospice. The cure is no longer possible. These patients are past the stage when the disease they suffer from will be cured. Of perhaps greater importance, though, is the fact they can be cared for, kept comfortable and out of pain, and measures can be taken to prevent the onset of social isolation. In these ways, hospice has demonstrated its worth, and hospice care has and will continue to be increasingly accepted by the public as an option for those whose life is coming to an end.

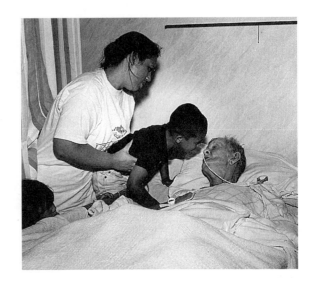

Figure 7-5 *Family members need to be involved in hospice care.*

HOME CARE

Health care delivery has gradually been moving away from the traditional hospital setting into more nontraditional arenas. Many changes in health care are a result of market-driven reform. In 1993, the U.S. Department of Commerce identified home health care as the fastest-growing segment of the health care industry (*U.S. News and World Report*, 1993). Respiratory home care is often a viable alternative to hospitalization. Chronic pulmonary disease is manageable in the home environment. A survey conducted by the American Association of Retired Persons found that an overwhelming majority of older adults would prefer home treatment over hospitalization (Bunch, 1996).

More long-term care patients are taken care of at home than in nursing homes. Over two million older people are cared for by home health care agencies each year (Dey, 1995). This figure represents about 7 percent of the elderly in the United States, whereas only about 4.1 percent of those 65 and older are residents in nursing homes at any one time. There are about 7,000 home health care agencies in the country, and older people represent about three-quarters of their patients.

The majority of their elderly patients are women. For both sexes, the use of home health care advances rapidly with age, from about 4 percent of those at age 65 to almost 15 percent of those age 85 and above. Over half of the women are widowed. By contrast, less than 20 percent of the males are widowers. The older women are more likely to live alone. Overall, men are much more likely to have a family member to care for them (Dey, 1995). Those who have family caregivers are less likely to enter nursing home care (Jette, Tennstedt, and Crawford, 1995).

Many older adults diagnosed with chronic bronchitis, emphysema, and other chronic airflow obstructive processes demonstrate chronic hypoxemia. Long-term oxygen therapy has been a widely accepted lifesaving treatment for these patients. In 1995 it was estimated that some 800,000 people were on home oxygen therapy in the United States (O'Donahue, 1995).

Home care can be short term for several months or long term for a year or for several years. The most important outcome of home care should be to improve the patient's quality of life. If by doing so the quantity of life is extended, then an additional benefit has been achieved. However, simply prolonging survival is not the principal goal.

INITIATION OF HOME CARE

Respiratory home care can be initiated as a result of an assessment in the physician's office. Most generally, home care follows an episode requiring hospitalization. Ideally, home care planning begins when the patient is admitted to the hospital. According to the American Hospital Association, discharge planning is a centralized, coordinated, interdisciplinary process that ensures a continuity of care for each patient (Lucas et al., 1988). When the patient is going to require home oxygen therapy or related respiratory care equipment, the respiratory care practitioner and the supervising physician should be responsible for overseeing that area of discharge planning. Based on the Clinical Practice Guidelines developed by the American Association for Respiratory Care (AARC), protocols are used by many home care companies. Documentation, or some type of form or checklist, must be filled out prior to the patient receiving home care. Patient information, a diagnosis, and a complete physician's order for therapy are required components. Many home care companies also have their respiratory care practitioners complete an initial patient assessment form, a patient care plan, and documentation of training for any equipment provided to the patient (Figures 7-6, 7-7, and 7-8).

For home care to be successful, an important underlying issue needs to be attended to: education. Patients and their families or caregivers must be trained on equipment and medication usage. The respiratory care practitioner needs to assume the role of an educator, a consultant, and a coordinator of care (Pierson, 1994).

Reimbursement.   Reimbursement for home care providers by third-party payers includes only the sale or rental of the equipment that is furnished to the patient. The Medicare Part B program that covers equipment does not now, and is not likely to in the future, reimburse for the services of a respiratory care practitioner (Dunne, 1997). Most home care companies are classified as durable medical equipment (DME) vendors. The DME vendors maintain respiratory care practitioners on staff, even though respiratory care is not a reimbursable service under Medicare. The services of the respiratory care practitioner are included as part of oxygen and equipment fees. Failure of the federal program to recognize and reimburse for professional respiratory care practitioner services has not, however, stemmed the growth of respiratory home care.

Hospital-based home care companies are providing an alternative that is gaining support from respiratory care practitioners and physicians alike. Hospital-based home care companies provide hospital-to-home service, a seamless continuum of care. Hospital-employed respiratory care practitioners provide training and education to the patient and

BROWN'S HOME HEALTH SUPPLY
14315 "C" Circle • Omaha, NE 68144
(800) 481-5744 • (402) 330-6406

HOURS:
Mon.-Fri. 8:00 to 5:00

Oxygen Training Certification

Patient Name: _____

Person Receiving Orientation: _____

Address:_____ Telephone: _____

Prescribed Therapy: _____ Liters/minute: _____ Hours/day: _____

Physician: _____ Referral: _____

Equipment Mfg. Model: _____ Serial No. _____ Hours: _____

Supplies: ❑ Cannula ❑ Mask ❑ Humidifier ❑ Tubing ❑ Other _____

GOAL: At the end of this training, the primary caregiver will be able to: 1) operate the oxygen system safely as prescribed, 2) understand the follow-up schedule to be maintained while the system is in the patient's home, and 3) replace D or E tank if applicable.

OBJECTIVE: To demonstrate an understanding of:
❑ The function and purpose of the oxygen equipment.
❑ How to adjust liter control knob or flowmeter.
❑ How to fill and attach humidifier, if required.
❑ How to clean and disinfect humidifier, if required. Vinegar Instruction Sheet left with patient (check here) ❑
❑ How to assemble and disassemble oxygen equipment. Replace D or E tank in cart if applicable.
❑ How to assemble equipment troubleshooting
❑ How patient/caregiver demonstrate all of the above via return demonstration to insure understanding.
  ❑ Oxygen booklet left with patient (check here)

❑ How to attach and use nasal cannula.
❑ When to use backup system

❑ How to use OCI device

SAFETY INFORMATION:
❑ Explain safety precautions and potential hazards of oxygen. Post NO SMOKING signs.
❑ Explain importance of following the physician's prescription. Advise patient to contact Brown's Home Health Supply if their prescription changes.
❑ Explain the importance of using distilled water in humidifier.
❑ Explain the importance of following humidifier cleaning procedures.
❑ Ask for questions or need for clarification.
❑ Explain approximate supply time of oxygen at prescribed rate, and oxygen delivery schedule.
❑ Give patient oxygen instruction materials, and Patient Bill of Rights & Responsibilities.
❑ Give patient telephone number for routine and emergency equipment situations.

LIQUID O₂ ONLY
❑ Explain the need for ventilation to prevent oxygen accumulation.
❑ Explain the effects of cold gas and liquid on skin and eyes.
❑ Explain that slow escape of gas through relief device is normal.
❑ Explain handling of portable LOX.
❑ How to read the contents gauge.
❑ How to fill portable unit.

CYLINDER O₂
❑ How to turn on cylinder. How to turn off cylinder when not in use.
❑ How to read pressure gauge.
❑ How to replace an empty cylinder, change regulator, or turn on manifolded cylinders, if required.

CONCENTRATOR ONLY
❑ How to understand audible alarm function.
❑ Explain the importance of audible power failure alarm
❑ Explain the importance of following humidifier and concentrator cleaning procedures.
❑ How to clean oxygen equipment. check and clean air inlet filter frequently.

NOTICE TO PATIENT: Your physician defines your treatment using the oxygen equipment. Brown's Home Health Supply and manufacturer assume no responsibility concerning the effectiveness of oxygen treatment of for the success or failure of nay treatment performed with the equipment. Should the equipment malfunction for any reason, call Brown's Home Health Supply. We will correct the problem or replace the equipment. Liability is limited to repair or replacement.

Comments: _____

Customer Signature: _____

Signature of Person Giving Orientation: _____ Date _____

8

Figure 7-6 *Oxygen training certification. (Source: Reprinted courtesy of Brown's Home Health Supply, Omaha, NE. Copyright 1996, Brown's Home Health Supply.)*

Patient Clinical Assessment and Follow-up

Patient Name: _____ Telephone: _____

Referral Physician name: _____ Referral _____

Diagnosis: _____

Equipment Ordered: _____ Prescription: _____

Equipment/Mfg.: _____ Serial Number: _____

Goals or Clinical Respiratory Service:
Equipment Management Goal: Will receive Brown's Home Health Supply follow-up visits to insure that the patient/client understands the safe operation of the equipment in the home care setting according to the physician's orders.
CARE PLAN: To insure that the patient/client understands the instruction received to safely operate the equipment in the homecare setting according to the physician's orders.

COMPLIANCE WITH CARE PLANS	YES	NO	NEEDS HELP
Patient understands and performs procedures well.	___	___	___
Patient understands emergency procedures and back-up systems.	___	___	___
Patient understands safety measures.	___	___	___
Patient understands infection control procedures/equipment is clean.	___	___	___
Patient has been treated for a respiratory infection since last visit	___	___	___
Patient understands routine maintenance procedures.	___	___	___
Home environment contains potential hazards or problems.	___	___	___

BP	
Pulse	
RR	

Physiological Parameters Assessment

Baseline SA02:	
With 02	
Without 02	
SA02 At Rest: With 02	
Without 02	
SA02 During ADL/Exercise With 02	
(Circle one) Without 02	

Medication: Amount/Frequency

Family Support/Environmental Conditions

Hospital Dates: _____

Date of Next Visit: _____

Psychological/Comprehension Assessment

Identified Problem/Need: _____

Goal: _____

Action Steps: _____

Plan: _____

Equipment Function: ☐ Acceptable ☐ Unacceptable **Back-up Oxygen System:** Size:_____ Amt in Tank _____ PSI
Concentrator Checks: _____ % at _____ LPM ☐ Flow Check ☐ Alarm Battery Model No.: _____
Filters Checked: ☐ Gross Particle ☐ Felt ☐ Bacteria Meter Hours:_____ Serial No.: _____

Patient/Caregiver Signature _____ Repspiratory Therapist_____ Date _____

Figure 7-7 *Patient clinical assessment and follow-up.* (Source: *Reprinted courtesy of Brown's Home Health Supply, Omaha, NE. Copyright 1996, Brown's Home Health Supply.*)

Patient Treatment Orders

Patient Name: _____ Date of Birth _____ Telephone: _____

Address: _____ City: _____ State: _____ Zip: _____

Primary Diagnosis: _____

Secondary Diagnosis _____

Prognosis: _____

Authorization for Clinical Respiratory Care Services

Dear Dr.:

Our records indicate that we have your patient in our respiratory clientele, if you wish to have any of the following performed on your patient, please check the appropriate boxes and return to our office in the self addressed stamped envelope provided. JACHO and the State of Nebraska requires that we have this prescription on file prior to doing any of the following. Thank you for your time!

Sincerely,

Craig Overman, Director
Brown's Home Health Supply

I wish to have the following performed on my patient by a licensed and credentialed respiratory therapist on a regular basis. This order is good for a period of one year.

❑ Breath Sounds, Heart Rate, Respiratory Rate, and General Assessment
❑ Pulse Oximetry on prescribed level of oxygen
❑ Pulse Oximetry on room air
❑ Routine instruction and follow up visits as needed

All of the above are preformed on a regular follow up visit "Free of Charge".

Signature: _____ Date: _____

Patient Care Plan

Patient's Problem or Need: ❑ Oxygen Therapy ❑ Altered Respiratory ❑ Altered Cardiorespiratory Function

❑ Other: _____

Goals:
   ❑ Will receive respiratory equipment supplies per physician's orders.
   ❑ Will be knowledgeable in equipment use and purpose of therapy.
   ❑ Will comply with physician's orders.
   ❑ Will use equipment safely in the home according to instructions.
   ❑ Will receive skilled respiratory care per physician's orders
   ❑ Other: _____

Care Plan:
   ❑ Provide equipment and oxygen therapy per physician's orders.
   ❑ Instruct in proper use and maintenance of equipment.
   ❑ Assess understanding and compliance with physician's orders.
   ❑ Deliver oxygen and supplies.
   ❑ Service equipment per service protocols.
   ❑ Provide skilled respiratory therapy per physician's orders above.
   ❑ Complete clinical record.

❑ Follow-Up Frequency: ❑ Monthly ❑ Quarterly ❑ Other _____

Consent: Patient has consented to the above plan of care?
   ❑ Yes ❑ No

Potential Problems: ❑ Infection control protocol
                  ❑ Potential environment hazards/precautions
                  ❑ Other _____

Continuing Care Review: (Date and Initial) 1. _____ 2. _____ 3. _____ 4. _____ 5. _____ 6. _____
                                    7. _____ 8. _____ 9. _____ 10. _____ 11. _____ 12. _____

Respiratory Therapist _____ Date: _____

16

Figure 7-8 *Patient treatment orders and care plan. (Source: Reprinted courtesy of Brown's Home Health Supply, Omaha, NE. Copyright 1996, Brown's Home Health Supply.)*

his or her family. They travel to the patient's home, set up equipment, do initial assessments, make follow-up visits, and complete follow-up patient assessments when needed. These same respiratory care practitioners are on call 24 hours a day for the patient. Whether it is to answer a question, troubleshoot equipment problems, or replace equipment, the patients receive personalized care. Many hospital admissions have been prevented by prompt and appropriate interventions by respiratory home care practitioners.

Managed care organizations are now appreciating the value of utilizing respiratory care practitioners in the home. Although there is an initial cost outlay, the cost benefit of employing respiratory care practitioners is favorable. Economically, home respiratory care makes sense. It has been estimated that the cost of 1 day in an acute care hospital is equivalent to the cost of 10 weeks of home respiratory care (Dunne, 1997). There are currently between 5,000 and 10,000 home care respiratory practitioners (Bunch, 1996).

A relatively new concept, **collaborative self-management,** is finding its way into respiratory home care. Patients are expected to assume a greater degree of responsibility for their medical condition. As the term implies, this concept depends on patients and health care professionals working together. The four elements of collaborative self-management are (Dunne, 1997):

1. Initial and ongoing assessment
2. Patient–caregiver education and training
3. Follow-up home visits
4. Consultative services

Home care respiratory care practitioners are in a unique position to enhance collaborative self-management (Make, 1995). Respiratory care practitioners have the training and knowledge to educate patients on self-management. Home care respiratory care practitioners are in the patients' homes on a regular basis and can perform assessments and work as consultants. As long as practitioners continue to upgrade their assessment skills, demonstrate expertise in the wide variety of home care equipment, and willingly serve as educators to patients and their families, respiratory home care will continue to grow.

Pulmonary Units.   Although many patients are very manageable in the home setting, some diagnoses and some types of equipment are more difficult to manage at home. A family support system for the home care patient is extremely important. When it is absent or nonfunctional, and when the patient is technology-dependent, pulmonary units in subacute or skilled nursing facilities are a reasonable alternative. Many patients no longer need hospitalization but still require mechanical ventilation. Most ventilator patients are transferred to postacute care settings after failure to wean in the hospital (Smirniotopoulos, 1994). Pulmonary units in postacute care are less formal, more homelike, and generally well tolerated by patients. Overall patient rehabilitation is the main goal. Often in this setting the emphasis on rehabilitation and the deemphasis on weaning enables recovery of ventilatory reserve in a surprisingly short period of time. Some patients are eventually weaned and leave the facility without ventilatory support. Respiratory care practitioners are well suited to this environment. A broad-based knowledge of pulmonary physiology, diverse clinical skills, and the ability to educate patients have made them valuable subacute care team members.

Health care in postacute care facilities holds great opportunity for respiratory care practitioners (Cornish, 1997). Postacute pulmonary care also makes good economic sense. It is less expensive than acute care and is billable to Medicare.

Home care, including hospice, visiting nurse service, and care by relatives, is usually seen as far preferable by the person concerned and his or her family. It is clearly the trend in the United States. Community-based programs for the aged see their goal as keeping people at home, out of institutions, for as long as possible. This trend may take the form of service delivery to the disabled individual—programs that are service extenders to the family. It is generally the case that whatever help that can be given to family caretakers saves costs over the long run.

RELATIONSHIPS WITH ADULT CHILDREN

Most older persons interact socially with family and friends on a regular basis. However, there remains a group of between 10 and 20 percent of the elderly who have little social contact with others, either family or friends. These isolated people usually have greater needs and are more likely to become institutionalized. Among those age 85 and above, Johnson and Troll (1992) found that there are widely diverse patterns of family interaction and help from adult children. Many in this group are widows and live alone; some have no surviving child living nearby. There is a risk among the oldest old of outliving their families. About one-third of those studied by Johnson and Troll had a family member serving as a caregiver; another 35 percent had someone available if help were needed. However, the remaining 29 percent had no one available to help them if they needed it.

Siblings and other relatives do not usually become substitutes for adult children or spouses when it comes to caregiving. Further, those older people living alone tend to be net receivers of support (Hirdes and Strain, 1995), which implies that people living alone are the most vulnerable.

In those situations where there is an available family member to serve as caregiver, it is most likely a spouse, and if a spouse is not available, an adult child. Being chosen (often by default) as the adult child who has caretaking responsibilities for the parents is frequently a source of resentment and family conflict.

In most instances, adult children who have the responsibility of helping an older parent say that they are glad to do it, and for the most part these are amiable relationships. However, increasing dependency on the part of the older person and little available help for the adult child caregiver can lead to strain and burnout, even abusive relationships.

The adult child responsible for parent care often feels stuck, and she may feel that she is unjustly burdened with more of the parental care duties than is her share. It is frequently the case that caretakers look to brothers or sisters for help and find little or none forthcoming. One typical study found that caregivers commonly seek more help than they receive (Karlin and Bell, 1992). Another study found siblings to be as much a source of stress as they were a source of help when parents needed care (Suitor and Pillemer, 1993). This research looked at 95 daughters providing care for demented parents; 195 members of social networks were also studied. It was found that the friends were at least as helpful as siblings. Brothers and sisters, on the other hand, not only were not of much help but it turned out that they were the most important source of interpersonal stress. Arguments over who should take responsibility for aspects of care, and resentment over those not taking their share, were frequent.

Abuse and Neglect.   Caregiver strain sometimes leads to abuse or neglect, especially when the caregiver receives no help. It is difficult to determine the actual prevalence of either abuse or neglect. Those who are abusive are unlikely to come forward, and those who are abused may be too embarrassed or fearful of retaliation to report it. Many incidents go unrecorded, and there usually is no central place or registry to gather information on cases of elder abuse. Conversely, instances where no actual abuse is present may be inappropriately recorded.

Pillemer and Finkelhor (1988) took a listing of all persons 65 and over in the Boston metropolitan area and took a stratified random sample of 2,813 of them. Only 63 out of the 2,020 who were interviewed had been maltreated in one way or another. A total of 40 had experienced physical violence, 26 had experienced chronic verbal aggression, and 7 were victims of neglect. Of those who reported physical violence, 45 percent had something thrown at them, 63 percent had been pushed, 42 percent had been slapped, and 10 percent had been hit, bitten, or kicked.

The most frequent category of abuser was wives (36.5 percent), followed by husbands (22.2 percent), sons (15.9 percent), daughters (7.9 percent), and others such as siblings or grandchildren (17.5 percent). The conclusion arrived at by the researchers was that a comparison of elder abuse to spouse abuse was more appropriate than a comparison to child abuse. More wives abused husbands in later years, however, indicating the direction of the caretaking responsibility.

Those living alone were much less likely to be abused—a rate only a quarter as high as those who lived with others. Widowed, divorced, and never married individuals were much less likely to be abused. Those in poor health were three to four times more likely to be abused, and males were much more likely to be abused physically and psychologically than were females. Females, on the other hand, were more likely to be neglected. Given the limits of their study, Pillemer and Finkelhor (1988) estimated that there are between 700,000 and a million abused older people in the United States.

Adult protective social workers are often called in where there are instances of apparent abuse, and the usual case they see is one of neglect. Financial abuse by adult children is probably the most common type of maltreatment of the aged. It is, however, hardly ever reported or brought to the attention of authorities. Often, abusers have a history of their own problems—frequently mental illness or alcoholism. One emerging group of offenders consists of children and relatives who take money from older people to support drug habits.

Stealing from older persons, especially from relatives, takes many forms. Nonpayment of loans probably involves the greatest actual dollar loss. Material abuse can be more common when older people have diminished capacity for management of their own financial affairs. In many cases, material abuse is committed by a relative or other caretaker who knows the older person well and has an opportunity. Larceny by strangers and con men makes the headlines, but material abuse by relatives no doubt occurs with greater frequency. Older victims are unlikely to complain.

The most common problem with older people who are not receiving proper care, however, might come under the heading of self-neglect. The model of the incapable caretaker who lashes out against a demanding, dependent older person, or whose incompetence results in neglect, might not always be appropriate. Instead, elder abuse and neglect might be better seen as a problem of a society where old people have little value because they are invisible.

Health care professionals must do what they can to report instances of obvious abuse or neglect. Much of the research on elder abuse points to the fact that dependent people in need of care are often a source of stress and strain to their caregivers, many of whom feel overwhelmed (Pillemer and Wolf, 1990). This research is in contrast to an earlier theory of family violence postulating that older people who are abused were themselves abusive parents. By this reasoning, the adult child harbors resentment and ultimately has an opportunity to get even. Those children who were abused in earlier life are not often the ones relied upon for caregiving. Spouses are much more likely to be caretakers of frail older people. Caregivers who do not receive help may reach the limits of their abilities and then either strike out or neglect the person for whom they are caring.

Patterns of family violence do exist, however, and one finding in the literature that is somewhat unexpected is the dual direction of violence. That is, violence by elderly people toward their adult children has gone unstudied for the most part. "The authoritarian father who ruled his children with an iron fist and dealt with a loss of authority or control by a beating apparently still resorted to these techniques at age 90. When the father found it to be more difficult to maintain control over children, he resorted to temper tantrums and physical outbursts" (Kosberg, 1983, p. 141).

The research gives practitioners an idea of what to look for in cases of abuse or neglect. Those identified in adult protective service records usually are females and have low incomes (Cash and Valentine, 1987), which may be due to the fact that financial strain is one of the most likely factors contributing to an overall pattern of stress in families. If the caregiver is running out of resources, money may be one of the most obvious resources. Other risk factors include advanced age and being dependent. High risk factors among caretakers include inexperience with caregiving, economic problems, and alcohol or substance abuse. Lack of family support and marital problems may also be present.

Combative or helpless older people might also be subject to abuse in nursing homes or other institutional settings. One study that interviewed 477 nurses and aides found that 10 percent admitted engaging in physical abuse and 40 percent in psychological abuse of patients. This behavior was often in response to patients who were themselves abusive (Pillemer and Moore, 1990). Again, the reasons given for patient abuse involve caregiver strain and lack of resources. The double direction of violence may also be present.

All fifty states have laws dealing with elder abuse and neglect. Emergency room personnel are increasingly being trained in the signs of abuse and the reporting requirements involved. Respiratory care practitioners may at times come across victims of physical abuse. They should consult their supervisors or others on the interdisciplinary health care team. It is often the physician or the social worker's responsibility to report cases of abuse, but any member of the team can raise questions about suspicious bruises, fractures, or malnutrition. Training family members on proper care techniques may help them in learning to better cope with a dependent elder.

IMPLICATIONS FOR RESPIRATORY CARE

The profession of respiratory care is intimately involved in geriatrics. Long-term care, either at home or within an institution, implies geriatric care. The growth of the older population and life-extending technologies indicates the increasing need for respiratory therapy in long-term-care and subacute care facilities (Chop, 1995). In fact, the trend is to move stable, long-term ventilator patients out of acute care hospitals into less expensive subacute care centers (Villa, 1994). Full-service respiratory care is also a growing ancillary service within skilled nursing homes (Wiedeman, 1994).

To date, much of the periodical literature in the field of respiratory therapy relevant to long-term care has dealt with two issues: the need for and growth of respiratory care for geriatric patients, and cost and reimbursement issues. What has not been emphasized is the variety of psychosocial needs of older people in long-term care. It is important for all health care and social service personnel to be aware of the messages received by chronically ill people who have increased their level of dependency. Imagine the loss of autonomy represented by the stark fact of not being able to get along at home anymore. Having decisions made by family members and health care professionals can promote a kind of sick-role behavior that leads to helplessness and a failure to thrive. People institutionalized against their will sometimes respond to this kind of loss by turning their faces to the wall and dying.

SUMMARY

Survival within long-term care demands involvement. Participation in decision making is vital if the elderly are psychologically to continue buying into the world of the living. Taking decision-making power away from people only serves to emphasize that they are no longer a full participant in this life. It is too easy, especially in respiratory therapy where people often have communication barriers, to simply provide mechanical care without inquiring as to what the patient's preferences are, or, indeed, without even talking to the patient.

Compassionate care means involvement in the activities of everyday life. The less people are involved in life, the less they will feel a part of it. Unfortunately, institutions by their nature tend to take people out of this everyday world into another, foreign place. Respiratory care practitioners need to constantly be aware of these barriers to living and do everything possible to eliminate them.

Review Questions

1. In what ways is home care less expensive than nursing home care?
2. Why are current nursing home patients described as being sicker than those of a generation ago?
3. Why do institutions tend to be regimented?
4. What are some signs of high social worth among patients?
5. Why is tracking the history of nursing home patients so difficult?

6. How does the hospice philosophy differ from ordinary long-term care?
7. Why do elders living alone have less potential for being abused?
8. Describe a situation in which respiratory home care would be beneficial to the older adult.
9. Discuss reasons why respiratory home care is not always ideal.

References

Bakwin, H. (1949). Emotional deprivation in infants. *Journal of Pediatrics, 35,* 512–521.

Blenkner, M. (1967). Environmental change and the aging individual. *The Gerontologist, 7,* 101–105.

Bourestom, N., and Tars, S. (1974). Alterations in life patterns following nursing home relocation. *The Gerontologist, 14,* 506–510.

Braun, J. V., Wykle, M. H., and Cowling, W. R. (1988). Failure to thrive in older persons: A concept derived. *The Gerontologist, 28,* 809–812.

Brody, E. M. (1985). Parent care as a normative family stress. *The Gerontologist, 25,* 19–29.

Bunch, D. (1996). Home care comes of age as health care moves outside of hospitals. *AARC Times, 20* (10), 18–27.

Cash, T., and Valentine, D. (1987). A decade of adult protective services: Case characteristics. *Journal of Gerontological Social Work, 10,* 47–60.

Chop, W. C. (1995). Resources for an aging population. *RT—The Journal for Respiratory Care Practitioners, 8* (1), 25–29.

Cornish, K. (1997). The respiratory care practitioner in extended care facilities. *Respiratory Care, 42* (1), 127–129.

Dey, A. N. (1995, March 20). Characteristics of elderly men and women discharged from home health care services: United States, 1991–92. *Advance data from vital and health statistics: no. 259.* Hyattsville, MD: National Center for Health Statistics.

Dunne, P. J. (1997). Respiratory care for the homebound patient. *Respiratory Care, 42* (1), 133–140.

Ellison, D. L. (1969). Alienation and the will to live. *Journal of Gerontology, 24,* 361–367.

Hirdes, J. P., and Strain, L. A. (1995). The balance of exchange in instrumental support with network members outside the household. *Journal of Gerontology: Social Sciences, 50B,* S134–142.

Holt (1897). *The diseases of infancy and childhood.* New York: Appleton.

Jette, A. M., Tennstedt, S., and Crawford, S. (1995). How does formal and informal care affect nursing home use? *Journal of Gerontology: Social Sciences, 50B,* S4–12.

Johnson, C. L., and Troll, L. (1992). Family functioning in late late life. *Journal of Gerontology: Social Sciences, 47,* S66–72.

Karlin, N. J., and Bell, P. A. (1992). Self-efficacy, affect, and seeking support between caregivers of dementia and non-dementia patients. *Journal of Women and Aging, 4* (3), 59–77.

Kosberg, J. I. (1983). *Abuse and maltreatment of the elderly: Causes and interventions.* Boston: John Right.

Kosloski, K., and Montgomery, R. J. V. (1995). The impact of respite use on nursing home placement. *The Gerontologist, 35,* 67–74.

Lefcourt, H. (1973). The function of the illusions of control and freedom. *American Psychologist, 28,* 417–425.

Lewis, M. A., Cretin, S., and Kane, R. (1985). The natural history of nursing home patients. *The Gerontologist, 25,* 382–388.

Liu, K., and Manton, K. (1984). The characteristics and utilization of pattern of an admission cohort of nursing home patients. *The Gerontologist, 24,* 70–76.

Liu, K., and Manton, K. (1991). Nursing home length of stay and spend down in Connecticut, 1977–1986. *The Gerontologist, 31,* 165–173.

Lucas, J., Golish, J., Sleeper, G., and O'Ryan, J. A. (1988). *Home respiratory care.* Norwalk, CT: Appleton and Lange.

Maizler, J. S., Solomon, J. R., and Almquist, E. (1983). Psychogenic mortality syndrome: Choosing to die by the institutionalized elderly. *Death Education, 6,* 353–364.

Make, B. (1994). Collaborative self-management strategies for patients with respiratory disease. *Respiratory Care, 39* (5), 566–578.

Montgomery, R. J. V., and Kosloski, K. (1994). A longitudinal analysis of nursing home placement for dependent elders cared for by spouses vs adult children. *Journal of Gerontology: Social Sciences, 49,* S62–74.

O'Donahue, W. J. (Ed.). (1995). *Long-term oxygen therapy.* New York: Marcel Dekker.

Pierson, D. J. (1994). Controversies in home respiratory care, conference summary. *Respiratory Care, 39* (4), 294–307.

Pillemer, K. A., and Finkelhor, D. (1988). The prevalence of elder abuse: A random sample survey. *The Gerontologist, 28,* 51–57.

Pillemer, K. A., and Moore, D. M. (1990). Highlights from a study of abuse of patients in nursing homes. *Journal of Elder Abuse and Neglect, 2,* 1–2, 5–29.

Pillemer, K. A., and Wolf, R. S. (1990). *Elder abuse: Conflict in the family.* Dover, MA: Auburn House.

Sirrocco, A. (1994, Feb. 23). Nursing homes and board and care homes. *Advance data from vital and health statistics: no. 244.* Hyattsville, MD: National Center for Health Statistics.

Smirniotopoulos, T. T. (1994). Subacute respiratory care: How to succeed at weaning without really trying. *Journal of Subacute Care, 1* (2), 4–7.

Strahan, G. W. (1997). An overview of nursing homes and their current residents: Data from the 1995 National Nursing Home Survey. *Advance data from vital and health statistics: no. 280.* Hyattsville, MD: National Center for Health Statistics.

Sudnow, D. (1967). *Passing on: The social organization of dying.* Englewood Cliffs, NJ: Prentice-Hall.

Suitor, J. J., and Pillemer, K. A. (1993). Support and interpersonal stress in the social networks of married daughters caring for parents with dementia. *Journal of Gerontology: Social Sciences, 48,* S1–8.

U.S. News and World Report (1993, April 26). The case for home care.

Villa, B. (1994, March). Subacute care centers. *Advance for Managers of Respiratory Care, 3* (2), 10–15.

Wiedeman, G. T. (1994). The growth of respiratory care at the skilled nursing facility. *AARC Times, 18* (5), 54–55.

CHAPTER EIGHT

THE END OF LIFE

KEY TERMS

activities of daily living
   (ADLs)
advance directives
DNR (do not resuscitate)

durable power of attorney
   for health care
euthanasia
living will

Patient Self-
   Determination Act
slow code

LEARNING OBJECTIVES

After completing this chapter, the reader should be able to:

1. Differentiate research findings on death anxiety among different groups.
2. Explain how care may differ according to the patient's perceived social worth.
3. Describe two types of advance directives.
4. Explain situations where cardiopulmonary resuscitation (CPR) is not appropriate.
5. Describe four categories of euthanasia.
6. Give details on the appropriateness of terminal weaning.
7. Name the group in society that is most likely to commit suicide.

INTRODUCTION

The term *geriatrics* implies not only old age but also death. Death in old age also implies chronicity; most of the people who die do so in late life, and most of the old people die over some length of time. Fewer than 20 percent of those who die in old age experience what could be called a sudden death. An important part of geriatric respiratory care includes caring for chronically ill older people whose illness will ultimately result in their death.

DEATH IN OLD AGE

The message of death is interpreted differently by younger people and older people. Certainly, there are very few people who wish to die. Most people do what they can to maintain life, and maintaining life is the foundation of respiratory care. Much of the respiratory care practitioner's orientation is on rehabilitation of those who will live for some time, or at least providing the means for people with respiratory disability to maintain life. Some of the efforts of practitioners—certainly the most dramatic ones—are in saving lives through interventions such as cardiopulmonary resuscitation.

However, death is not always the enemy. This is a difficult concept, particularly for those whose orientation is in saving life at almost any cost. Those whose lives are extended do not always receive this extension as a gift that is appreciated. Perhaps the differences in meanings of death can be clarified with a review of some of the research on attitudes toward death.

DEATH ANXIETY

As part of a continuing series of studies, Thorson and Powell (1988) surveyed 599 adolescents and adults with a death anxiety scale. They found that females as a group were slightly but significantly higher than males in fear of death. A much greater difference, however, was by age. Young people were much more afraid of death than older people. At first this seemed to be a paradox: Why should those closest to death—the aged—fear it the least? Another question raised from these data was related to the first finding. Women outlive men by almost 7 years, on the average. If they live longer, why should they have greater death anxiety than men?

Looking at the various elements of death, it was determined that women tended to express greater fears of pain and bodily decomposition. Young people were significantly more likely to fear not only decomposition but also the perceived immobility associated with death, the uncertainty of what happens after death, the pain associated with death, helplessness, isolation, and loss of control. In contrast, the fears associated with death that were higher among the aged dealt mainly with the uncertainty of an afterlife and what the next world would be like.

This survey led to a hypothesis that death anxiety and religiosity might be related, especially for those who seemed to have greater concerns about the afterlife. In another study, Thorson and Powell (1990) tested 346 people, ranging in age from 18 to 88, with the death anxiety scale as well as a scale designed to measure intrinsic religious motivation. One explanation for lower death anxiety among the aged might be a result of the life review, a process of reminiscence brought on by a realization of impending death. The life review is a way people reflect on the meaning of their lives and come to terms with who they are and what they have done in life. Perhaps those who have completed a life review have a better religious understanding as well. The data supported the hypotheses that both age and religiosity associate negatively with fear of death. Older people scored significantly higher on intrinsic religious motivation and lower on death anxiety than young people. Those who scored higher in religiosity were lower in fear of death, and those higher in death anxiety were lower in religiosity.

An interpretation from these and other studies of death anxiety is that older people may fear death, but they fear it less than young people. They might sense death's inevitability. They have lived their lives, they see others their own age dying around them, and they begin to realize that their own time is approaching. They seek to find a sense of resolution concerning the meanings of both life and death (Figure 8-1). Their fears tend to be mainly associated not with death itself but with the discomfort associated with the process of dying.

Elisabeth Kubler-Ross (1969) has said that the greatest fear that dying people have is of isolation, of being left alone at the very end. Dying people, especially dying older people, are often perceived as being so low in social value as to be virtually invisible. Health care professionals need to guard against patients becoming ignored and isolated at the very end.

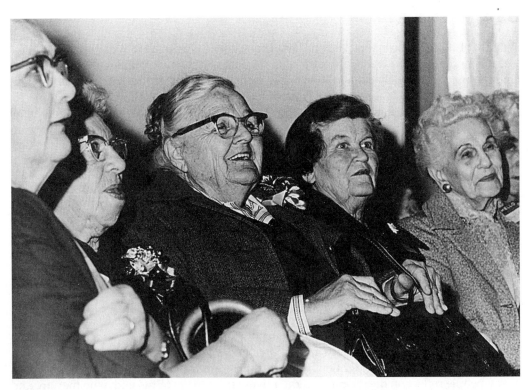

Figure 8-1 *Many older people have resolved anxieties associated with death.*

DEMOGRAPHY OF LIFE AND DEATH

Most of the people who die are old people (Table 8-1). According to the discussion in the first chapter of this book, the increase in life expectancy is explained for the most part by the fact that a larger proportion of the society is living out the greater potential of their allotted time. Over three-quarters of white men and 86.7 percent of white women live into old age. The racial differential in longevity is pronounced, but it is diminishing. The gap used to be wider between white and black; it will continue to narrow. Among the oldest old, women have a remarkable probability of living into extreme old age: 42.5 percent of white women and 30.5 percent of black women live at least until age 85.

FUNCTIONAL STATUS

The functional status of very old people, while limited, is not always severely restricted as death approaches. The proportion of men and women who are fully functional decreases, and those who are severely restricted increases during the last year of life (Table 8-2). The

TABLE 8-1 Chances per 1,000 of Surviving to a Specific Age

Age	White	Black
Males		
15	987	975
25	973	948
35	957	909
45	931	846
55	881	749
65	763	592
75	546	389
85	238	150
Females		
15	990	980
25	985	972
35	979	958
45	968	929
55	939	875
65	867	766
75	712	576
85	425	305

Source: *Metropolitan Life Insurance Company.* Statistical Bulletin, *July–September, 1993, p. 31. Reprinted by permission.*

TABLE 8-2 Percentages of Fully Functional and Severely Restricted Decedents, by Age at Death, Sex, and Type of Preexisting Condition

Preexisting Condition*	Age at Death					
	65–74		75–84		85+	
	Men	Women	Men	Women	Men	Women
Fully Functional						
Hypertension	28.6	17.8	15.4	12.9	7.9	4.4
Heart disease	27.4	18.3	17.7	14.8	10.8	4.0
Cancer	38.0	9.3	12.7	15.9	9.3	0.0
Stroke	15.2	5.8	2.2	4.5	1.8	1.6
Lung condition	19.2	11.8	13.2	9.1	4.8	3.3
Diabetes	20.8	18.1	11.3	12.2	12.1	1.4
None	23.2	16.6	19.3	11.0	13.1	5.6
Severely Restricted						
Hypertension	2.5	4.6	5.3	12.3	12.3	21.0
Heart disease	0.4	4.7	5.5	9.2	9.2	21.7
Cancer	0.0	0.0	4.2	13.8	24.8	22.8
Stroke	4.2	13.3	17.5	23.4	30.8	39.1
Lung condition	0.9	6.4	5.8	9.9	4.9	23.0
Diabetes	2.8	8.1	7.4	14.0	20.2	24.2
None	0.5	4.7	4.0	14.0	9.7	26.6

*A preexisting condition is defined as a condition that existed 12 months prior to death and that was not the underlying cause of death. Categories are not mutually exclusive.
Source: *H. R. Lentzner, E. R. Pamuk, E. P. Rhodenhiser, R. Rothhenber, and E. Powell-Griner (1992). The quality of life in the year before death.* American Journal of Public Health, 82, 1096.

activities of daily living (ADLs) are generally restricted for most people as they approach death, but they are not totally restricted. That is, many older people, even in their last year of life, can still do things for themselves—eat, dress, and bathe themselves, get up and go to the bathroom without help, and so on. The proportion who are fully functional goes down with advancing age. For example, of women who die of heart disease between the ages of 65 and 74, 18.3 percent are fully functional in their last year of life. This declines to 14.8 percent at ages 75 to 84, and to only 4 percent by age 85. Chronicity and disability increase with age.

Those who are severely restricted, however, do not represent a mirror image of those reported in the fully functional category. Taking women who die from heart disease as an example again, only 4.7 percent of those ages 65 to 74 are severely restricted. This percentage increases with age to 21.7 percent by age 85. It can be inferred that there are quite a few in a middle ground; they are neither fully functional nor severely restricted. They have some impairments in their ability to accomplish the activities of daily living, but they are not totally restricted in what they are able to do. Those who have had a stroke are the most likely to be severely restricted and least likely to be fully functional. The ones with severe restrictions are, of course, those most likely to need therapeutic care and are most likely to be seen by respiratory care practitioners.

Implications.   Very old people are sometimes starved for touch, they often perceive themselves to be low in social value, and they are the most likely people to become isolated (Figure 8-2). Special efforts need to be made not only to keep them involved in society but also to give them reassurances that they are not being abandoned. Taking time to sit and listen, hold a hand, talk, remember in any way—all of these efforts are much appreciated. Therapy goes beyond the mechanics of setting up lines or pumps. A good interpersonal relationship with patients is an ideal to work toward, no matter how sick or disabled they might be.

TYPES OF DEATH

Guarding against social death will mean a personal, rather than a mechanical, relationship with patients. Unfortunately, the likelihood of social death occurring depends on many

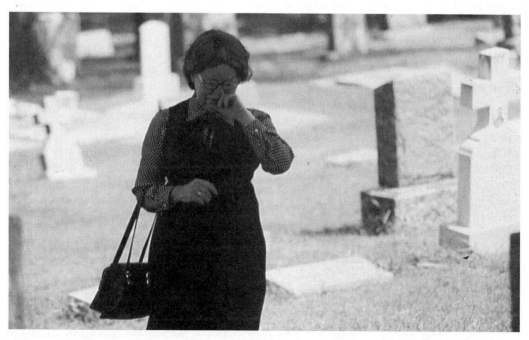

Figure 8-2   *Grief and loneliness, particularly for widows, contribute to a sense of isolation.*

things. It is natural to find some patients to whom it is easier to relate. The type of death or the underlying condition, however, is also an important variable. Those who are unresponsive are the ones with whom it is hardest to develop a personal relationship.

SOCIAL MESSAGES

Rapport goes beyond ascribed social value or attractiveness. Sudnow (1967), for example, found that very poor and very unattractive patients were the least likely to get much interpersonal care. He found that alcoholics and drug addicts were looked on judgmentally by medical staff. Sudnow was writing before the era of acquired immune deficiency syndrome (AIDS). Perhaps he might have found strong staff attitudes toward people with AIDS had he been writing on social death in the 1990s rather than the 1960s. Research indicates, for example, that men with AIDS exhibit much higher levels of covert death anxiety compared with other terminally ill men (Hayslip, Luhr, and Beyerlein, 1992). Perhaps they detect an effort to create social distance among some of their caregivers. At least one study (Sweeting and Gilhooly, 1992) has found that social death tends to become more likely in three instances: when people are in their final stages of terminal illness, when they are very elderly, or when they have lost their essential personhood because of coma or dementia. The social message of the disease people are dying of might be added to this list.

Regardless of one's orientation to professionalism, nuances of attitude no doubt slip through in some instances, and social messages can be picked up by almost any lucid patient. The point is that there are a host of things that may determine the ability of the practitioner to develop and maintain good relationships with the dying. The ability to communicate certainly is one of those things. It is difficult to maintain much of a conversation with an individual who is comatose or on a ventilator. Special efforts must be made to talk to people who cannot respond.

Staff Attitudes.   We might think that cause of death would not have much influence on our feelings toward patients, but this is often the case. Imagine, for example, the differing attitudes staff members might have toward people who are equally disabled by, say, an accident or a drug overdose. To take another example, a gang member who has been shot and is dying presents a much different social and psychological message to health care professionals than does a young mother dying of septicemia. The alcoholic who has already had a liver transplant and who has continued drinking so that he is dying of cirrhosis is likely to engender much different feelings among his caretakers than a 95-year-old who develops congestive heart failure.

DIFFERENCES BY GENDER AND RACE

Types of death differ somewhat by gender and race. There are varying ratios of causes of death for men and women and blacks and whites (Table 8-3). For example, the male-to-female ratio for deaths from heart disease is 1.88 to 1.0. Males are 1.88 times more likely than females to die of heart disease. Blacks are 1.48 times more likely than whites to die of

TABLE 8-3   Ratio of Age-Adjusted Death Rates for 15 Leading Causes of Death for the Total Population by Sex and Race: United States, 1992

Rank Order	Cause of Death (*Ninth Revision, International Classification of Diseases*, 1975)	Ratio of— Male to female	Black to white
1	Diseases of heart	1.88	1.48
2	Malignant neoplasms, including neoplasms of lymphatic and hematopoietic tissues	1.45	1.37
3	Cerebrovascular diseases	1.18	1.86
4	Chronic obstructive pulmonary diseases and allied conditions	1.70	0.81
5	Accidents and adverse effects	2.63	1.27
	Motor vehicle accidents	2.35	1.03
	All other accidents and adverse effects	2.97	1.57
6	Pneumonia and influenza	1.69	1.44
7	Diabetes mellitus	1.14	2.41
8	Human immunodeficiency virus infection	6.97	3.69
9	Suicide	4.28	0.58
10	Homicide and legal intervention	3.98	6.46
11	Chronic liver disease and cirrhosis	2.42	1.48
12	Nephritis, nephrotic syndrome, and nephrosis	1.53	2.76
13	Septicemia	1.28	2.71
14	Atherosclerosis	1.33	1.08
15	Certain conditions originating in the perinatal period	1.22	3.21

Source: *National Center for Health Statistics,* Monthly Vital Statistics Report, 43, *(6),* Supplement, *March 22, 1995.*

heart disease. Interestingly, African Americans are less likely than whites to die of chronic obstructive pulmonary disease, by a ratio of 0.81 to 1.0.

For most of these causes, one might argue that differences are fairly innocuous. A heart disease patient probably does not engender much difference in staff attitudes than, say, a cancer patient or a stroke patient. However, there are several causes of death that are likely to cause potent differences in feelings of the health care team.

Males (particularly young males) are 2.35 times more likely to die in an automobile accident than females. It would be difficult not to have an attitude toward a young man who, under the influence of alcohol, was admitted to the hospital dying and who had perhaps caused the deaths of others in an automobile accident. Similarly, males are 4.28 times more likely than females to die from suicide. Staff members may have strong feelings about trying to save the life of someone who has made a deliberate effort to lose it. To not sit in judgment of patients oftentimes takes considerable maturity on the part of the practitioner. It is not easy to maintain the mindset that people are not good or bad; health care professionals need to work with people where they are.

At one time it was emphasized in professional training that one must "keep a stiff upper lip," maintain a certain distance, and not get personally involved with the lives of patients. This kind of old-fashioned attitude ignores practical considerations. It is almost impossible to not get involved in people's lives—and it also ignores the fact that human empathy is often what makes the difference in quality care. Practitioners should not be afraid to form friendships and show warmth and genuineness with the people they care for. Bereavement for patients who die is natural and normal. Practitioners should take the time to discuss their feelings with others on the staff when a person they have become close to dies.

QUALITY OF LIFE ISSUES

Dying is not a pleasant experience for most people, but it is not often the stuff of horror stories. The quality of life in the last year depends on a number of things. It obviously depends on the underlying medical condition. No one wants to be disabled and helpless for a period of weeks or months prior to the end. Age is another factor, in addition to illness, that contributes to the quality of life or lack of it. One recent study, for example, points to persons with human immunodeficiency virus (HIV) infection. A total of 369 individuals were tested with a variety of measures. It was demonstrated that the oldest ones had significantly poorer ratings in medical outcomes such as physical function, health perception, role function, social function, and mental health. Older subjects, however, reported less pain (Piette et al., 1995).

PAIN

Pain is the principal variable identified as the thing feared most about the process of dying. In the realm of pain management, however, there are contradictory studies of the same population by the same authors. The first (Lawton, Moss, and Glicksman, 1990) followed 150 terminally ill older patients and 200 of their relatives. It was reported that 82 percent of the persons who died experienced a generally positive quality of life over the course of their final year. It was concluded from these data that most people die peacefully.

In a follow-up with the 200 surviving relatives, however, it was found that pain had increased over the final year. By 1 month prior to death, fully two-thirds of the terminally ill patients had felt pain frequently or all of the time. Pain, not surprisingly, contributed significantly to lower happiness and greater levels of depression (Moss, Lawton, and Glicksman, 1991). It is difficult to reconcile these studies because of the conclusions. Two-thirds being in pain much or all of the time during the final month does not contribute to a message of peaceful death.

There is a lesson here on patient advocacy. The respiratory care practitioner is not the individual in charge of medical care. However, any professional dealing with a patient can ask questions. If a person is in constant, obvious pain, it is incumbent upon professionals to see if relief can be provided.

CASE STUDY: ON WATCHING AN OLD MAN DIE

Jerry, an old friend, called one evening to tell me of the frustration he was having with the hospital care received by his 85-year-old father. His dad had emphysema and congestive heart failure; he'd been in a nursing home for 3 months. When he had a respiratory arrest there, they sent him to the hospital. Now he was in the intensive care unit, there was a tube down his throat, he was barely clinging to life, semiconscious, and the doctors wanted to do a tracheostomy—to cut a hole in his throat and put the old man on a ventilator.

I asked Jerry if he knew that once his dad was on the ventilator there would be little chance of ever getting him off of it. He did. Then I asked him why they wanted to go ahead with the procedure on a man who was so obviously at the end of his life.

"Well, he went into the nursing home 3 months ago, and they had him fill out a **living will**," Jerry said. "On it, there was an item asking if he wanted to be resuscitated if the situation arose, and he checked it off, saying that yes, he did want it."

The doctor at the hospital took that as an **advance directive** that Jerry's father wanted all available means used to keep him alive. I asked Jerry if that was what he thought his father would, in fact, have wanted. No, he didn't think so. In fact, he was sure that he specifically did not want to spend his last weeks or months with a machine breathing for him. Several times he had already tried to pull out the tubes that were in his nose and mouth.

"So," I told him, "First thing in the morning, you go and meet with the doc. Tell him you are the person responsible for your father, that the situation has changed since he was in the nursing home, that you do not authorize him to go ahead with the surgery, and that you want only comfort measures for your father. If he gives you any trouble, tell him you have power of attorney. (Jerry did in fact have power of attorney for his father's financial affairs, but he didn't have a specific **Durable Power of Attorney for Health Care**.) He won't ask to see it. If you want someone to go with you to meet with the doc, I'm willing."

He thought he could handle it without having me along. I told him not to be surprised if his dad lingered on for a few more days.

This was on a Sunday night. That next Thursday I got a call from Jerry's wife. She said the medical staff had been only too willing to go along with Jerry's request; they'd actually been waiting to hear something from the family to prevent what they thought would probably be a useless procedure. Jerry's father was out of intensive care, he was in a regular hospital room, his daughters were in from out of town, and everyone was reconciled to this being the end of his life. Only their son was going to perform in his last high school program that evening, and they'd like to go see him. . . .

I picked up on where that was going. "And you don't want Dad to die alone," I said. "What time should I be there?"

So I took a stack of term papers with me to grade and went over to the hospital that evening to sit with an old man while he died.

He was lying there on his back with his mouth open, puffed up like a blister from the congestive heart failure, obviously close to the end. His breathing was labored, short little

Source: James A. Thorson (1995). *Aging in a changing society.* Belmont, CA: Wadsworth, pp. 337–339. Reprinted by permission.

puffs that weren't doing him any good. He wasn't conscious, but he wasn't quite comatose, either. Jerry told me earlier that his dad hadn't been able to recognize him or respond to him for some time. When I went over and took his hand to tell him who I was, one eye did open for a moment. It didn't focus on me, but it did open. And he squeezed my hand.

As I sat there next to him, reading my papers, it was clear that he wouldn't be able to keep breathing like that for much longer; he would die of exhaustion. I timed him. At 7 P.M. he was taking 23 breaths per minute; at 8 P.M. it was up to 30. By 9 P.M. he was taking 43 breaths per minute. I shouldn't say breaths; they were pants. Try taking 43 breaths per minute and see what I mean.

There was a monitor hooked up to him; the top number gave his blood oxygen levels, the bottom his pulse. He had an oxygen tube in his nose and an intravenous line giving him saline or glucose. Respiratory therapy people came in twice while I was there to give him some help and to suction the gunk out of his trachea. I turned off the TV; it seemed to be just one final indignity to have to die to a *Matlock* rerun. When the monitor indicating his heartbeat slipped below 50, the light would turn from green to red, and a beeping noise would sound. I asked the nurse if she could turn down the volume of that, as the noise seemed to agitate him.

"But if I turned off the sound, we couldn't hear it."

"That's right. It's all right if you don't hear it."

She understood, and she turned off the sound. She agreed that all that was wanted now was comfort measures and that he had "DNR" written on his chart. In other words, we were in an open awareness; the man was dying, it was all right, and they wouldn't do cardiopulmonary resuscitation on him when he finally did die.

On the other hand, he was still hooked up to an antibiotic drip. Damned if I knew just what good that was going to do.

The reading on both monitors gradually slipped down and down; the pulse monitor was red much of the time now, reading in the 40s for the most part. His breathing became even more labored, if possible. The first time both monitors went flat and read zero, I figured that was it. The old man continued to pant along, though, and I began to have less faith in electronic monitors and more in the basic human instinct to cling to life. The monitors went down to zero several more times while I was still on shift.

Jerry and his sister came in to relieve me late that evening; they'd enjoyed the program at the high school and were most appreciative. The old man died at 1:00 that morning.

He wanted a Dixieland band at his funeral. He got it.

The point of the case study is that it integrates much of what has already been said with much of what remains in this chapter. The old gentleman had signed an advance directive, which is discussed in the next section. It was unclear to the medical staff exactly how that directive was to be interpreted, which is fairly typical. They were going to go ahead with the aggressive course of treatment, against their better judgment, which may also be fairly typical. Had the son not mustered the courage to act as his father's advocate, the story may have had an unhappy ending: The patient might have lived.

This flies in the face of everything given as an orientation to health careers. The ending was happy because the patient did *not* live. This was not a case where the patient was simply old and thus unimportant. The extra mile was in fact about to be taken by the physician despite the fact that the course of treatment really would not lengthen life so much as draw out the course of death. Social value in this instance actually had little to do with decision making. Jerry knew his father's wishes, he knew his father's life was over, and he knew that further efforts not only would be futile but downright harmful.

One might surmise that the father had little fear of death, but he was confused when a form for his signature was thrust in front of him at the nursing home. If he had been a person with no family, the form he signed would have sentenced him to life on a ventilator in some quiet ward of warm bodies in subacute care. Respiratory care practitioners would shake their heads as they went about their business, wondering why in the world someone thought that keeping his poor old body alive was contributing to his life. It should be pointed out that this case was real and it happened just a few years ago. Also, it is not a particularly unusual case.

ADVANCE DIRECTIVES

Note that the case study made mention of durable power of attorney for health care, which is a type of advance directive. In this instance, it is a document appointing another individual to take charge of decision making if the patient is unable to make decisions for himself. The other type of advance directive is a living will, a statement giving directions on how the patient wishes to be treated in the event that he or she can no longer communicate. Both the durable power of attorney for health care and the living will give the patient some control over what will happen in terms of treatment at the very end of life.

The use of these documents grew out of increasing concern with the possibilities of modern technology keeping people alive—against their will—for some period of time after their lives are in fact over. Many people are reacting to horror stories they have heard about people being preserved in a vegetative state. In fact, many of these cases are of people who either have no one to speak for them because they have no family members or the family cannot be reconciled to the reality that their loved one's life is over.

CASE STUDY

Robbie was hit by a car on his way to school and had extensive brain damage. He was comatose for 3 months and then unexpectedly regained consciousness in the hospital. He was not able to talk, but he did draw pictures, could smile, and it was evident that he could understand what was said to him. His family had been praying for a miracle, and it looked like their prayers were being answered.

Then, something happened. The details are a little sketchy, depending on who is questioned, and because memory changes a bit over the years. The best that can be determined is that Robbie went into respiratory arrest and his monitor was either not properly hooked up or was defective in the way it worked. At any rate, when he finally was found and resuscitated, he was profoundly damaged, in a deep coma. For a while, who to blame was a consideration, but it was clear that it was the hospital that had the deep pockets. Suing a nurse or a therapist would not get very far. The hospital quietly came to an accommodation with the family. The care costs that were not paid by Blue Cross would be absorbed by the institution, not billed to the family.

The hospital, of course, did not know that Robbie would be taking one of their ICU beds for another 12 years. His mother spent every afternoon there. She was devoted to the thought that her little boy would be up and running again some day and refused to believe otherwise.

Robbie had, and was cured from, seemingly every infection that passed through the intensive care unit over the years. Nurses and therapists quietly spoke of the resentment of staff who felt that resources were being squandered on a hopeless case, all because of a mother who could not grasp the reality that her son was in fact dead, that his body merely was being sustained in a kind of quasi-state of life. Others spoke of the ambivalent feelings of Robbie's brothers, who felt they had not only lost a brother but also a mother.

Finally, when the million-dollar limit on the Blue Cross policy was nearly reached, a pulmonary subacute care unit opened in a local nursing home. Robbie was transferred there. He died 11 months later. He had been in a coma for 13 years.

This case study proves that advance directives are not always the solution in every case, desirable as they might be. In this instance, a minor child would not be expected to have a living will or a person appointed with durable power of attorney for health care. It would be assumed that his parents would make decisions, which they did. That their decisions did not please everyone was to be expected. No doubt they anticipated another miraculous return from limbo for Robbie. At what point—in the fifth month or in the fifth year—did it become apparent to almost everyone else that this was a vain hope? It is almost always easier to not make a decision. In this instance, doing nothing meant maintaining the status quo; doing something would have meant a decision to terminate life-sustaining measures.

Here there are a host of ethical and legal problems. Letting someone die goes against the grain, and removing the means by which life is sustained is even more difficult. Further, problems of liability are uppermost in the minds of the administrators of health care institutions. The fear of being sued has made many a doctor and many a hospital go to seemingly absurd degrees in extending treatment.

THE PATIENT SELF-DETERMINATION ACT

The **Patient Self-Determination Act** was mandated by the federal Omnibus Budget Reconciliation Act of 1990 (Madson, 1993). It underlines the patient's basic right under the law to refuse treatment. Every health care program—hospital, nursing home, or home health care agency—that receives federal funding must provide information to newly admitted patients, giving them the opportunity to designate someone to speak for them if they become unable to speak for themselves. It also gives them the option to make a statement of the circumstances in which they do or do not wish to have life-sustaining treatment. In essence, it allows patients to create a living will or to appoint someone to have durable power of attorney for health care.

Institutional Variations.   The phrasing of these statements under the Patient Self-Determination Act varies from one institution to another. Further, specific wording of accepted forms for a living will or appointment of an individual to have durable power of attorney for health care may be different from one state to another. For respiratory care practitioners, no doubt the orientation given by staff development departments for new employees should cover these specifics. If it does not, *ask.* For patients, a copy of the particular form can be obtained on request from the health care institution and should be provided with admission materials. Additionally, the specific form acceptable in any particular state to make a living will or to appoint another person to have durable power of attorney for health care can be obtained by writing to Choice in Dying, 250 West 57th Street, New York, NY 10107.

The document prepared by a hospital or other health care institution is often seen as being quite formidable by patients, particularly by the elderly and especially by those being admitted under crisis circumstances. Heart attack and stroke victims being admitted through the emergency department of a hospital, for example, may not comprehend the specifics of the document. Staff should be trained to carefully explain the implications of possible modes of care. Unfortunately, circumstances for patient education are hardly ever ideal. The individual may be confused or may not understand just what a particular phrase or paragraph really means.

This situation is found in the first case study in this chapter. Jerry's father, when admitted to the nursing home, simply checked off that he wanted all available means used to sustain life. When the implications of this option are explained, many patients react in horror: "Oh! I don't want to be kept alive on a lot of tubes and machines!" Yet, few people have taken the effort to plan and execute these kinds of documents prior to when they will be needed.

In other circumstances, an advance directive is not useful if (1) there is no one to appoint—those without family or close friends, for example; (2) the individual is essentially looking to the health care provider for assisted suicide; or (3) the individual is confused or comatose and it is too late to execute a valid document.

Nevertheless, advance directives provide some comfort to patients, and to health care providers and institutions as well. A clear, unambiguous living will can give the medical staff guidance on the limits of treatment that are wanted. A person with terminal cancer might quite properly sign a statement indicating that he or she does not wish to be resuscitated. The same message might be conveyed by a person authorized to speak for the patient. Having an individual with durable power of attorney for health care gives the staff one designated person to speak to. Problems of multiple family spokespeople are thus avoided.

There is little doubt that advance directives are needed. One recent study looked at the last 3 days of life among a sample of 1,227 elderly persons (Foley et al., 1995). Family members were interviewed 3 months after the event. Most of the people who died did so either in a hospital (45 percent) or a nursing home (24 percent). About a third knew that death was imminent, but in almost half of the cases death was unexpected. Forty-four percent of the patients had difficulty recognizing family members at the very end. Fifty-three percent died in their sleep. Many had failed to discuss their wishes with relatives.

Another study surveyed 1,000 older people. Eighty-five percent felt that people should have the right to request the withholding or withdrawal of life-sustaining treatment, but only 12 percent had completed any kind of advance directive document (Luptak and Boult, 1994). This study went on to detail methods by which trained volunteers and social workers counseled elderly patients and their families on the exact meaning and implications of advance directives. In this instance, 71 percent then went on to complete an advance directive and 96 percent of these named a proxy for decision making.

Health care staff have less anxiety on how a patient should be treated when a clear statement of intent has been made. In many situations, unless "no code" is written on the patient's chart, staff members are duty bound to make efforts at resuscitation with whatever means are available. This action sometimes seems inappropriate to staff, and anyone who has been employed in a health care institution for even a few years has heard war stories about the patient who was resuscitated twelve times in 2 days. Instances of a **slow code** might circulate in the grapevine of communication. A slow code is the situation in which calling the CPR team seems futile but must be done. Resuscitation is attempted only after the patient is "good and dead," so the efforts at bringing the individual back to life are guaranteed to be unsuccessful.

THE SUPPORT PROJECT

The Robert Wood Johnson Foundation has funded many research projects on the care of patients nearing death. The SUPPORT (Study to Understand Prognoses and Preferences for Outcomes and Risks of Treatments) project was one such effort (SUPPORT Principal Investigators, 1995). A 2-year prospective observational study with 4,301 patients was followed by a 2-year controlled clinical trial with 4,804 patients and their physicians. This trial was divided into an intervention group of 2,652 and a control group of 2,152 patients in five teaching hospitals in the United States. These were people with diagnoses of life-threatening illnesses; the overall 6-month mortality rate was 47 percent. Particular efforts were made with the intervention group to educate the patients and their family members and improve understanding of outcomes, encourage attention to pain control, and facilitate advance care planning.

Results of the project were disappointing. In the first phase, only 47 percent of physicians were aware that their patients had executed an advance directive. About half of **do-not-resuscitate (DNR)** orders were written within 2 days of death. Thirty-eight percent of patients who died spent at least 10 days in intensive care. Family members reported that over half of the patients who died had moderate to severe pain at least half the time. There were no improvements in the second phase of the project. The authors concluded, "Enhancing opportunities for more patient–physician communication, although advocated as the major method for improving patient outcomes, may be inadequate to change established practices" (1995, p. 1,591). A companion editorial to the SUPPORT project report in the *Journal of the American Medical Association* stated:

SUPPORT documented serious problems with terminal care. Patients in the study experienced considerable pain: one half of patients who died had moderate or severe pain during most of their final three days of life. Communication between physicians and patients was poor: only 41% of patients in the study reported talking to their physicians about prognosis or about cardiopulmonary resuscitation (CPR). Physicians misunderstood patients' preferences regarding CPR in 80% of cases. Furthermore, physicians did not implement patients' refusals of interventions. When patients wanted CPR withheld, a do-not-resuscitate (DNR) order was never written in about 50% of cases. (Lo, 1995, p. 1,635)

In other words, a concerted effort in five major hospitals over the course of 4 years, at the cost of millions of foundation dollars, was a total failure at getting physicians to recognize patients' basic rights under the Patient Self-Determination Act. Perhaps doctors were too busy to consider end-of-life issues among their patients. This finding pointed to the serious need for patient advocacy on the part of all health care practitioners.

APPROPRIATENESS OF CARDIOPULMONARY RESUSCITATION

The research has a number of studies wherein CPR efforts clearly are futile. A study by Applebaum, King, and Finucane (1990), for example, sought to determine outcomes following attempted cardiopulmonary resuscitation initiated in nursing homes by ambulance crews called to transport them to hospitals. This study included 705 people age 65 or over. Possible outcomes included death in the emergency room, death during subsequent hospitalization, or live discharge. Only two lived longer than a few days. One who survived was an 87-year-old woman who spent 30 days in the hospital and died 8 months after returning to the nursing home. The other was an 81-year-old man who returned to the nursing home after a 60-day hospitalization and died there 14 days later. "We conclude," the authors say, "that the benefits of cardiopulmonary resuscitation initiated in nursing homes are extremely limited" (1990, p. 197).

The implications of this study are disturbing. Is CPR among the very old ineffective? Is it merely a way to drag out the process of dying? Clearly, many of these people had reached the end of their lives, and the efforts at resuscitation were something of a ritual drama, grasping at one last straw prior to accepting the inevitable. Perhaps CPR has become an obligatory step to take before finally admitting that the individual indeed is dead.

It might also be questioned why ambulance crews had been called to resuscitate nursing home patients. One might surmise that nursing home staff had not been trained to do it themselves. There is no information from this study on the rate of success of CPR efforts that were initiated by nursing home care staff members. One cynical way of looking at these data is that perhaps nursing home staff were in a sense passing the buck by calling an ambulance crew to care for a person in cardiac or pulmonary arrest. They were then not obliged to take care of the dead body, nor was the death recorded as having taken place in their facility.

There are a number of studies of CPR that were done within hospitals, rather than by ambulance crews called to households or to nursing homes. The first one presents data gathered in twenty-four hospitals in eight different countries over the course of 10 years: The Brain Resuscitation Clinical Trials I and II (Rogove et al., 1995). A total of 774 patients who were initially comatose after successful resuscitation had a 6-month mortality rate of 81 percent. For those age 80 and above, it was 94 percent, compared with a rate of 68 percent for those younger than 45 years of age. Twenty-seven percent of the patients recovered good neurological function. Independent predictors of mortality included a history of diabetes, arrest time of greater than 5 minutes, a history of congestive heart failure, a noncardiac cause of arrest, and a resuscitation effort of over 20 minutes.

The second study was of 255 events of cardiorespiratory arrest in a noncritical care area of a veterans' hospital (Berger and Kelley, 1994). Immediate survival was 52 percent. Survival after intensive care unit stay was 22 percent, survival to hospital discharge was eleven percent, and survival to follow-up 22 months later was 4 percent. It was noted that the post-CPR hospital charges for each of the surviving patients was estimated at an average of $63,000. Ten people (out of 255) were still alive 2 years later. It should be noted that these were patients in a noncritical care unit, not cardiac care, intensive care, or emergency room patients.

Perhaps it would be instructive to cite a brief portion of a recent review article (Hammill, 1995) that hearkens back to the origins of CPR:

> Cardiopulmonary resuscitation (CPR), as we know it, was introduced by Jude, Kouwerhoven, and Knickerbocker in 1960 for victims of acute insults such as drowning, electrical shock, drug reaction, anesthetic mishap, heart block, and dysrhythmias associated with acute myocardial infarction. They addressed indications and contraindications in this way: "Not all dying patients should have cardiopulmonary resuscitation attempted. Some evaluation should be made before proceeding. The cardiac arrest should be sudden and unexpected. The patient should not be in the terminal stages of a malignant or other chronic disease, and there should be some possibility of a return to a functional existence. The rigid time limit of 3 to 5 minutes since the onset of arrest of cardiac output should not be exceeded. In regard to the latter when there is a genuine question of the duration of arrest, resuscitation should be attempted." (p. 516)

Unfortunately, the author observes, current practice often appears to fail to meet such criteria. With the widespread training of health care providers and the lay public, CPR has come to be used for virtually anyone found in a pulseless state, unless documentation exists that the patient should not be resuscitated. Survival rates, however, have not improved dramatically since the 1960s. Initial success with resuscitation ranges from 30 to 50 percent. Hammill notes that survival to discharge occurs in about 15 percent of resuscitated patients. Of the survivors, between 10 and 20 percent have evidence of neurologic dysfunction. "Thus, many patients undergo cardiopulmonary resuscitation that results in an expensive prolongation of life but with no impact on the ultimate outcome" (1995, p. 515).

Implications.   It is clear that serious discussion needs to take place among members of the interdisciplinary health care team about the intent and ultimate effectiveness of various types of life-sustaining treatment. Persons in advanced stages of illness that probably will result in the termination of life, especially the very aged, often are not good candidates for resuscitative measures. Extending a life of pain, or being the cause of months or even years of irreversible dementia or neurological deficit, is not doing the patient or the family a favor. Extra efforts need to be made to not only educate older patients about the implications of their decisions under the Patient Self-Determination Act but also about what life-sustaining measures mean for family members.

TERMINATION OF LIFE SUPPORT

Ending efforts to sustain life presents ethical problems that go beyond the scope of this text. Removing food, hydration, or ventilator supports that sustain life—or removing any means that might support life—can be exceedingly difficult.

EUTHANASIA

Part of the difficulty in this ethical realm is confusion over what constitutes **euthanasia.** There are four different categories of euthanasia: combinations of active versus passive and voluntary versus involuntary.

Active Voluntary Euthanasia. Active voluntary euthanasia means killing someone at his or her request. Active euthanasia is an intentional intervention to end life. In the eyes of the legal system, a bullet to the brain or an overdose of morphine differ little if the intent was to kill the recipient, even if the person was pleading for death. Part of the Hippocratic Oath taken by physicians states, "Neither will I administer a deadly poison to anyone, even at his own request."

Some critics of Dr. Jack Kevorkian, the retired pathologist who has been prosecuted in Michigan for assisting terminally ill people to commit suicide, would say that actively injecting the solution that will kill, or merely providing it and letting the person flip the lever that will end his life, are essentially the same thing, that calling something "assisted suicide" rather than premeditated homicide is quibbling. It is important to note, however, that Kevorkian has never been charged with murder and that all of the people he has assisted have sought him out for help. Nor has he been convicted in any of the instances in which he has been prosecuted.

Active Involuntary Euthanasia. Active involuntary euthanasia is actively taking the life of a person who has not requested it, and it is usually seen as less ethically justifiable than active voluntary euthanasia. The individual actively taking another's life has taken it upon himself to determine who shall live and who shall die. Those responsible for active involuntary euthanasia are vulnerable to prosecution for murder.

Passive Voluntary Euthanasia. Passive voluntary euthanasia means letting a life end at the individual's request without intervention. The person who discovers that she has cancer of the pancreas and opts to have no treatment other than painkillers is in essence choosing passive voluntary euthanasia. She knows that the disease will kill her within a matter of weeks or months, there is almost no chance of a cure, and any medical efforts made to arrest the cancer will be painful, disfiguring, and probably futile. Is this the same as suicide?

Probably not, if the individual is in fact well informed of the odds and the circumstances of her illness.

Passive Involuntary Euthanasia.   Passive involuntary euthanasia means not being informed, and in some ways it is the least defensible of the four euthanasia categories from an ethical point of view. Letting someone die without his full knowledge or without even presenting him with his options seems particularly cold, but it often is a necessity when decisions for unresponsive patients must be made by others.

CASE STUDY

The professor of an undergraduate university course in death and dying discusses ethical choices with students. Many of the students are registered nurses seeking a degree. A few years ago, a student confessed something in class discussion. She had a patient, an aged woman in advanced stages of terminal cancer, who was pleading for death. The nurse knew that the woman had only a few days to live. The medication order for this patient included a certain amount of morphine to be titrated over 6 hours in a drip. The nurse said that she instead gave the woman the entire dose in one injection. The patient died 20 minutes later. The other nurses in the class were then asked how many of them had either done the same kind of thing or knew of it being done in a place where they had worked. About half of the hands went up.

ETHICAL DILEMMAS

The distressing thing about ethical problems is that there seem to be so few absolutes. The difference between one thing and another is neither white nor black, but instead comes in various shades of gray. Is rowing one's boat past a drowning man without saving him the same as killing him? Certainly, not saving a life in crisis cannot be morally defensible. However, what if the person jumped off the bridge? Does that make it a different set of circumstances, or is the issue still the same? To use an analogy closer to home, if a person who is already within a few weeks of death develops pneumonia, should it be treated? If a person with cancer of the spine has a burst appendix, is an appendectomy appropriate? Is it all right to let the person die of peritonitis? These are not easy questions to answer. More difficult yet are issues of withdrawal of treatment. The ethical and moral problems here are very difficult. A general principle is to save lives with the means that are available. Some ethicists would argue that letting someone die for, say, lack of hydration seems almost worse in some circumstances than administering an overdose and getting it over with.

CASE STUDY

A woman had a mother whose small-town general practitioner told her that her melanoma was inevitably fatal, that any treatment would be futile, and that she should go home and die. Her daughter wanted a second opinion, got her mother registered at one of the nation's major cancer centers, and the woman responded well to treatment, adding a dozen quality years to her life.

In the case study, the general practitioner thought he knew what was best for the patient. Taking his advice would have led to the woman's untimely death. Leaving people uninformed, either through ignorance or knowing better than they do, is not defensible. Deciding to let someone die without her consent is in some ways equivalent to taking life into one's own hands.

Removal of Life Supports. Removal of life-sustaining means can involve very difficult moral decisions. Removing life supports involves a number of different dimensions. Not feeding or hydrating a person, for example, may be a far different thing than not doing coronary bypass surgery. Giving a person who is terminally ill food and water but withholding medications that may extend life may seem to be contradictory. If they are to be allowed to die of infection, why not cut off their water and get it over with? Treatments sometimes seem to be at cross-purposes. In this chapter's first case study, Jerry's father was "no code"—that is, when he died the official intention was to let him be dead. However, he did have an intravenous antibiotic drip, which seems fairly foolish in retrospect.

Unfortunately, a situation that is not discussed and examined is often rife with foolish and contradictory things. Family members and interdisciplinary health care members—and patients—need to address issues of life or death up front.

TERMINAL WEANING

Perhaps the situation where the respiratory care practitioner confronts these issues head-on most often is when it is decided to remove a patient from ventilator support. Whether or not to give CPR in the absence of an existing order is more of an instantaneous decision that is generally made by the attending nurse rather than the respiratory care practitioner. Once the CPR team is summoned, a crisis atmosphere is created, and in the rush it is very difficult to pause and say, "Now wait—does this patient really want to be resuscitated?" Instead, most people react instinctively, regardless of whether doing CPR is a good idea, and plow on ahead, doing what they have been trained to do. Thus, the vast majority of people who have CPR live for another day or two at best.

Removing a person from a ventilator, on the other hand, is generally a decision that has been arrived at after some consideration—it is not done in a crisis atmosphere. Only in the relatively few instances when such withdrawal is done without the knowledge or consent of the patient or family does this present a genuine moral and legal problem (Snider, 1995). In fact, decisions to remove ventilator support are made on a daily basis—mostly without much controversy—and often they represent a relief to everyone involved. When a therapy becomes futile, it is not wrong to withdraw it.

This may be all well and good from a hypothetical point of view; however, it often is a much different matter for the individual who does the hands-on work. Unlike turning off the ventilator as one might with a brain-dead patient, terminal weaning is a complex process (Campbell, 1994). In some instances, a patient who is not expected to live after being weaned from mechanical ventilation does continue to live, and in these instances sedation might reduce his or her chances of survival. Campbell (p. 38) presents a number of important points on terminal weaning:

1. How long the weaning will take depends on the patient. An unconscious patient generally may be weaned in less than an hour; a conscious patient usually requires more time.
2. One way to wean from the ventilator is to gradually reduce the minute volume of ventilation by reducing the rate. This produces hypercapnia and causes carbon dioxide narcosis, minimizing patient distress.
3. During rate reduction, one may need to adjust the FIO_2 (fraction of inspired oxygen). If the patient is hypoxemic and distressed, increasing the FIO_2 may reduce his distress. If he is neither hypoxemic nor distressed, consider decreasing the FIO_2 after reducing the minute volume. A patient can be hypoxemic but not distressed; intervene only if distress occurs.

Generally, signs of distress may be minimal if the patient is in deep coma. Sedatives should be provided for conscious patients, and the procedure should be under the supervision of a senior staff member. Sedation might contribute to an earlier death. Vincent and Lammers (1995) argue that this is similar to the situation in which large doses of narcotics are given to patients with terminal cancer—the treatment of the pain may well hasten the individual's death—which usually is exactly what the individual has in mind. Their explanation is that this sedation exemplifies the concept of "double effect," which justifies an action or omission if the following criteria are satisfied (p. 1,174):

1. One does not will the evil outcome, for example, the narcotic sedation is given to relieve the dyspnea and pain, not to kill the patient.
2. The act itself is not evil; there is nothing in itself morally wrong in refusing a treatment or using a narcotic to control pain or discomfort.
3. The good does not follow directly from the evil; for example, it would be wrong to kill a person in order to relieve his dyspnea; the evil of killing results in the relief of his suffering.
4. There is a proportional good involved. The dyspnea or feeling of suffocation is severe and causes great pain, suffering, and anxiety, which is relieved by the narcotic sedative.

SUICIDE

A total of 2,305,000 people died in the 12-month period ending September 1996. Of them, 29,830—about 1.3 percent—killed themselves (National Center for Health Statistics, 1997). Among all causes for all groups, suicide is the ninth leading cause of death. This statistic is deceptive, however, in that self-destruction is much more likely in some groups than in others. Demographically, the ratio of suicidal deaths between males and females is 4.28 to 1. That is, men are more than four times more likely to kill themselves than women. Between white and black, the ratio is 1.0 to .58—African Americans are much less likely to commit suicide than whites (Kochanek and Hudson, 1995).

DEMOGRAPHIC DIFFERENCES

The real demographic difference in suicide figures comes with the factor of age (Table 8-4). The group in American society that commits suicide the most is older white males (McIntosh, 1992).

Suicide is a major public health problem among older white men. Contrary to accepted stereotype, teenagers do not commit the most suicides in the United States. As a group, their rate of suicide is less than that for the population as a whole. The high social value of young people tends to make their suicides more newsworthy. An old man shooting himself is not the stuff of headlines. As a general rule, the suicide rate for females at any age is never half as high as the corresponding rate for males of the same age and race. The rates for African Americans at most ages are significantly lower than those for whites. The rates for women, both black and white, increase until middle life and then decline somewhat among the older age groups. Among black women, there are so few suicides in later life that the numbers do not meet statistical standards for reliability. This is also true for black males age 85 and older. The suicide rate for white males remains relatively stable across the middle adult years. It then increases dramatically in late life. The rate for older white men is eleven times higher than the rate for older white women.

TABLE 8-4   Suicide Rates by Sex, Race, and Age Group

Age	Total[1]	Male White	Male Black	Female White	Female Black
All ages[2]	12.2	21.7	12.1	5.2	1.9
10 to 14 years old	1.5	2.4	2.0	0.8	(B)
15 to 19 years old	11.0	19.1	12.2	4.2	(B)
20 to 24 years old	14.9	26.5	20.7	4.3	1.8
25 to 34 years old	15.2	26.1	21.1	5.8	3.3
35 to 44 years old	14.7	24.7	15.2	7.2	2.9
45 to 54 years old	15.5	25.3	14.3	8.3	3.0
55 to 64 years old	15.4	26.8	13.0	7.1	2.1
65 to 74 years old	16.9	32.6	13.8	6.4	2.4
75 to 84 years old	23.5	56.1	21.6	6.0	(B)
85 years and over	24.0	75.1	(B)	6.6	(B)

B = Base figure too small to meet statistical standards for reliability of a derived figure.
[1]Includes other races not shown separately.
[2]Includes other age groups not shown separately.
Source: 1994 Statistical Abstract of the United States.

GERIATRIC SUICIDE

Why do old white men commit suicide at such high rates? One explanation might be that the most stressful time of life for women comes in the middle years, while it comes in young adulthood for African American males and in later years for white males. The most accepted explanation of motivation for suicide is anomie. From a sociological point of view, anomie is defined as normlessness, social instability resulting from a breakdown of standards and values. Psychologists, on the other hand, would understand anomic behavior as a tendency to view the future with pessimism and to feel controlled by hostile outside forces—alienation resulting from helplessness and a lack of purpose in life. One study of geriatric suicide points to the primary motivation as being a desire to escape from intolerable life circumstances (Courage et al., 1993).

Much of the research points to an association of suicidal behavior with depression, and it is accepted that suicidal motivation often comes in wavelike patterns, coming and going in varying degrees of intensity. Perhaps older white males are the most likely group to have enjoyed an internal locus of control during adult life, whereas women and African Americans have been more likely to have been externally controlled. Old age may bring real prospects of a loss of control for older white males, leading to depression, helplessness, and isolation. The vision of being controlled by others, such as caregivers, may be seen as intolerable. This situation is especially true for those who have few social supports and who have lost their confidant through widowhood.

Older men tend to use more lethal methods of killing themselves and they are also more likely to use multiple means, which is an indication that they really do want to die, not just demonstrate a cry for help. In one study of suicide among old men, it was found that 85 percent used a gun, and in 65 percent of the cases the death was due to a gunshot wound to the head (Miller, 1978). Fewer than 5 percent in that study had taken drugs or inhaled lethal gas—means that are more characteristic of those who are ambivalent as to whether or not they really wish to die.

PASSIVE SUICIDE

Not everyone who wants to end life goes about it directly. Suicide statistics are thought to underestimate the actual number of deaths from self-destructive behaviors. Many accidents, for example, might have resulted from a suicidal motivation. Passive suicide—letting oneself die—goes unreported. Passive suicide can be seen among those who refuse to eat, who try to pull out their tubes, who alter or "forget" their medications, or who forgo treatment (Courage et al., 1993). Those who have given up the will to live may show clear signs of wanting to end life. This behavior does not necessarily have to be so obvious as the kidney dialysis patient who opts to discontinue treatment. Signs may be seen among the diabetic who binges on candy or who continually misplaces her insulin, or in the person with emphysema who continues to smoke. Many people are indifferent as to whether they wish to continue living. These people may be very difficult patients for the respiratory care practitioner—they may actively resist or resent treatment.

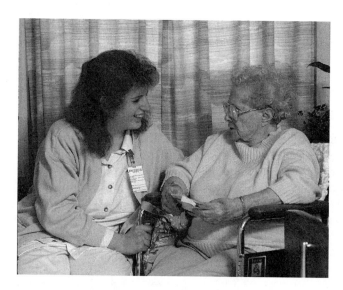

Figure 8-3 *Warm human relationships break down the forces of isolation.*

SUMMARY

Respiratory therapy in geriatrics often means working with the dying. Terminally ill people have the same needs as everyone else. Perhaps their greatest fear is isolation. Being left alone to die is all too common. Medical care staff and members of the general public are alike in that their attitudes predict behavior—their fear of death is often translated into an avoidance of the dying. Sudnow (1967) noticed that interaction with dying people decreased as they got closer and closer to death. Visits from friends and relatives dwindled off, the time given to them by their physician declined dramatically, and the number and length of contacts with nursing staff went down proportionately.

However, dying people themselves have testified that maintaining human contact is one of their greatest needs. Keeping people comfortable in their final weeks and days is a principal goal of care of the terminally ill. Any health care professional can act as an advocate for a patient who is in pain. Avoiding unnecessary and discomforting procedures is also important. Few people enjoy being prodded, stuck, poked, or intubated when there is little purpose remaining for the procedure in question.

Maintaining dignity and autonomy are also important goals. People do not appreciate being talked about in their presence as if they were not there. The sense of hearing is the last to go, and there are reports of people who have emerged from coma who could repeat conversations that were held at their bedsides. Persons who have been resuscitated have been able to testify as to what was said by whom during the procedure. Treating dying people with dignity should come as a matter of course. Maintaining patient autonomy means letting people make decisions for themselves. When or whether to do a particular procedure might be a decision best left to the person receiving it. Finally, good care demands that patients never feel abandoned.

Life-extending technologies are not always appreciated. Maintaining patient autonomy means respecting people's wishes as to whether, or in what circumstances, they wish to continue living. Patients need to have their options explained to them so that they can make intelligent decisions. If the time for patient decision-making is past, a proxy or advocate may have been appointed. The decisions of someone holding durable power of attorney for health care have the same weight legally as the patient's own decisions would have had in the same circumstances.

It is possible for any member of the interdisciplinary health care team to form relationships, even close bonds, with patients. Especially among the aged terminally ill, these friendships are much appreciated. It is quite possible that some patients have outlived all of their family members, that they have become isolated and alone. Health care personnel may be the only kind faces they see from day to day. It is incumbent upon practitioners to treat them with compassion, wisdom, and warmth as their lives come to a close.

Review Questions

1. Why do young people have the highest death anxiety?
2. Have you observed instances of better care given to persons of higher perceived social value?
3. In what instances is CPR not appropriate?
4. If doctors ignore living wills, what good are they?
5. How might passive involuntary euthanasia actually seem worse than active voluntary euthanasia?
6. What are some of the best ways to minimize isolation among older terminally ill patients?
7. How might durable power of attorney for health care be superior to living wills?

References

Applebaum, G. E., King, J. E., and Finucane, T. E. (1990). The outcome of CPR initiated in nursing homes. *Journal of the American Geriatrics Society, 38,* 197–200.

Berger, R., and Kelley, M. (1994). Survival after in-hospital cardiopulmonary arrest of non-critically ill patients. *Chest, 105,* 872–878.

Campbell, M. L. (1994). Terminal weaning. *Nursing 94, 24* (9), 34–39.

Courage, M. M., Godbey, K. L., Ingram, D. A., Schramm, L. L., et al. (1993). Suicide in the elderly: Staying in control. *Journal of Psychosocial Nursing, 31* (7), 26–31.

Foley, D. J., Miles, T. P., Brock, D. B., and Phillips, C. (1995). Recounts of elderly deaths: Endorsements for the Patient Self-Determination Act. *The Gerontologist, 35,* 119–121.

Hammill, R. J. (1995). Resuscitation: When is enough, enough? *Respiratory Care, 40,* 515–519.

Hayslip, B., Luhr, D. D., and Beyerlein, M. K. (1992). Levels of death anxiety in terminally ill men: A pilot study. *Omega: Journal of Death and Dying, 24,* 13–19.

Kochanek, K. D., and Hudson, B. L. (1995). Advance report of final mortality statistics, 1992. *Monthly vital statistics report,* vol. 42, no. 6, suppl. Hyattsville, MD: National Center for Health Statistics.

Kubler-Ross, E. (1969). *On death and dying.* New York: Macmillan.

Lawton, M. P., Moss, M., and Glicksman, A. (1990). The quality of the last year of life of older persons. *Milbank Quarterly, 68* (1), 1–28.

Lo, B. (1995). Improving care near the end of life: Why is it so hard? *Journal of the American Medical Association, 274* (20), 1634–1636.

Luptak, M. K., and Boult, C. (1994). A method for increasing elders' use of advance directives. *The Gerontologist, 34,* 409–412.

Madson, S. K. (1993). Patient Self-Determination Act implications for long-term care. *Journal of Gerontological Nursing, 19* (2), 15–18.

McIntosh, J. L. (1992). Epidemiology of suicide in the elderly. *Suicide and Life-Threatening Behavior, 22,* 15–35.

Miller, M. (1978). Geriatric suicide: The Arizona study. *The Gerontologist, 18,* 488–495.

Moss, M. S., Lawton, M. P., and Glicksman, A. (1991). The role of pain in the last year of life of older persons. *Journal of Gerontology, 46,* P51–57.

National Center for Health Statistics (1997, April 24). *Monthly vital statistics report,* vol. 45, no. 10. Hyattsville, MD: Public Health Service.

Piette, J., Wachtel, T. J., Mor, V., and Mayer, K. (1995). The impact of age on the quality of life in persons with HIV infection. *Journal of Aging and Health, 7,* 163–178.

Rogove, H. J., Safar, P., Sutton-Tyrrell, K., Abramson, N. S., et al. (1995). Old age does not negate good cerebral outcome after cardiopulmonary resuscitation: Analyses from the brain resuscitation clinical trials. *Critical Care Medicine, 23,* 18–25.

Snider, G. L. (1995). Withholding and withdrawing life-sustaining therapy. *American Journal of Respiratory and Critical Care Medicine, 151,* 279–281.

Sudnow, D. (1967). *Passing on: The social organization of dying.* Englewood Cliffs, NJ: Prentice-Hall.

SUPPORT Principal Investigators (1995). A controlled trial to improve care for seriously ill hospitalized patients. *Journal of the American Medical Association, 274* (20), 1591–1598.

Sweeting, H. N., and Gilhooly, M. L. (1992). Doctor, am I dead? A review of social death in modern societies. *Omega: Journal of Death and Dying, 24,* 251–269.

Thorson, J. A., and Powell, F. C. (1988). Elements of death anxiety and meanings of death. *Journal of Clinical Psychology, 44,* 691–701.

Thorson, J. A., and Powell, F. C. (1990). Meanings of death and intrinsic religiosity. *Journal of Clinical Psychology, 46,* 379–391.

Vincent, J. E., and Lammers, S. E. (1995). Ethics and patient care. In D. R. Dantzker, N. R. MacIntyre, and E. D. Bakow (Eds.), *Comprehensive respiratory care.* Philadelphia: W. B. Saunders.

GLOSSARY

ACE inhibitors angiotension-converting enzyme inhibitors. Act by suppressing renin-angiotension-aldosterone system, causing a decrease in blood pressure.

activities of daily living (ADLs) abilities that indicate the functional capacity of frail persons, such as dressing oneself, bathing, getting in and out of bed, walking, and getting to the bathroom without assistance.

activity theory the point of view that the best way to grow old is to remain active, to replace roles and functions lost due to old age with new ones.

advance directives a Living Will or a Durable Power of Attorney for Health Care stating the individual's wishes as life terminates.

affective disorders mental or emotional illness without an organic cause; depression is the most common of the affective disorders.

agammaglobulinemia a total deficiency of the plasma protein gamma globulin. This condition may be transient, congenital, or acquired.

ageism prejudice against older people.

age normative appropriate to one's age.

alpha$_1$ antiprotease a plasma protein produced in the liver that inhibits the activity of trypsin and other proteolytic enzymes.

Alzheimer's disease a chronic, fatal, neurological deterioration characterized by senile plaques on the brain and neurofibrillary tangles found on autopsy. Alzheimer's is probably the most common organic cause of dementia in later life.

aneurysm a balloonlike swelling in the wall of an artery.

angioplasty reconstruction of a blood vessel.

anomie hopelessness, feeling controlled by hostile outside forces, and viewing the future with pessimism.

arteriosclerosis a common term used to describe a group of diseases characterized by thickening, loss of elasticity, and calcification of arterial walls.

ascites an abnormal accumulation of fluid in the peritoneal cavity.

aspiration pneumonia pneumonia caused by aspiration of fluid or a foreign body.

atelectasis absence of gas from a section of the lung due to failure of expansion or reabsorption of gas from the alveoli.

atherosclerosis   a common arterial disorder associated with an accumulation of cholesterol, lipids, and cellular debris along the inner walls of the arteries.

atopic   an inherited tendency to develop allergic reactions.

autoimmune response   an autoimmune response is the body not recognizing part of itself
and responding as if there were a foreign invader; arthritis is an example of an autoimmune response.

backward failure   heart failure in which the cause is associated with passive engorgement
of the systemic venous system.

bacteremia   presence of live bacteria in the circulating blood.

beta-agonist   pharmacological agent that stimulates the beta receptor and has numerous
effects on the airway.

bioavailability   the portion of the administered dose of a drug that reaches the systemic
circulation.

biological clock   a genetic program for human fibroblasts to double about fifty times and
then cease; in a broader sense, it is a biological program for the organism to develop, mature, and then to ultimately fail.

biotransformation   a series of chemical alterations of a compound occurring within the
body.

bipolar disorder   an affective disorder characterized by alternating periods of mania and
depression.

carcinogen   a substance or agent associated with an increased incidence of cancer.

cardiorhexis   a rupture of the heart wall.

centenarians   those who have lived to age 100.

cerebrovascular accident (CVA)   a stroke; an occlusion of the blood vessels of the brain,
resulting in ischemia of the brain tissue.

Charcot-Brouchard aneurysm   small aneurysms found on tiny arteries within the brain of
elderly and hypertensive subjects.

chemoreceptor   a sensory nerve cell activated by chemical stimuli.

Cheyne-Stokes breathing   an abnormal breathing pattern characterized by a rhythmic
waxing and waning in the depth of respiration, followed by a period of apnea.

closing capacity   closing volume plus residual volume.

closing volume   the volume of gas in the lungs in excess of residual volume that remains
when small airways in the dependent lower portions of the lungs close during maximal
exhalation.

collaborative self-management   the patient and practitioner working together to assist in
making home care therapy possible.

community-acquired pneumonia   pneumonia that occurs in individuals who are ambulatory and living in a noninstitutional environment. Causative agents are usually pneumococcus and *Haemophilus influenzae.*

compression of morbidity   concentration of chronic and disabling conditions in the last
few years of life.

confidant   someone in whom you can confide.

continuity theory   the concept that old age is merely an extension of middle age, that people do not change very much as they get older in terms of their social needs.

cor pulmonale   an enlarged right ventricle of the heart due to pulmonary hypertension, secondary to diseases of the lungs or pulmonary arteries.

cross-linking theory   the concept that aging is caused by cellular cross-linkages and the accumulation of collagen in the tissues.

cumulation   the rate of drug elimination is slower than the rate of administration, causing a potentially toxic condition.

cytosol   the cytoplasm minus the mitochondria and endoplasmic reticulum components.

demography   the statistical study of human populations.

disengagement theory   the idea that aging is developmental and that old age is a genuinely separate period of life; it is characterized by a mutual separation of people from their former roles and society from needs for the older person. The disengaged person retires to the rocking chair and is happy about it.

DNR   do not resuscitate, an order to not initiate CPR in the case of circulatory or respiratory arrest.

drug duplication   use of more than one drug with the same pharmacological properties.

Durable Power of Attorney for Health Care   a signed statement appointing another individual to be responsible for making decisions on care, especially terminal care.

dyskinesia   an impairment of the ability to voluntarily control muscular movements.

dysphagia   difficulty in swallowing.

elastase   an enzyme that speeds up the breakdown of elastic tissue.

empathy   knowledge gained from having had the same experience as another.

endocrine theory   the concept that biological aging in the cells is regulated by hormones.

epidemiology   the statistical study of disease.

error catastrophe theory   the concept that DNA ultimately gives wrong messages for cell replication until a catastrophic error kills the organism.

euthanasia   terminating life, either directly or through the removal of life supports.

evolutionary model   genetically controlled repair ceases after maturation, as there is no evolutionary necessity for the organism to survive after reproduction.

exchange theory   the concept that there is mutual interchange between the generations, that help and services are traded off roughly equally; when inequality comes into the relationship, adult children care for their parents out of a sense of obligation and a realization of past services received from their parents.

failure to thrive   a progressive decline in functioning, including loss of weight, depression and listlessness, and decreased immune response.

febrile   relating to an elevated body temperature.

filial obligation   the feeling, not unlike guilt, that family loyalty has its demands; we should care for older relatives because we are supposed to care for family members.

first-pass effect   the first pass of a drug through the liver, in which hepatic metabolism takes place.

free radical theory   hydroxyl ions that are a product of metabolism seek to combine at the molecular level, causing damage that results in the aging of the organism; these ions may be controlled by antioxidants.

genetic program   the concept that maturation, system failure, and death of the organism are controlled genetically.

GERD gastroesophageal reflux disease. A disease caused by reflux of stomach contents into the esophagus.

geriatrics clinical care of the aged.

gerontology the study of aging processes.

granuloma a mass or nodule formed in response to chronic infection, or a chronic inflammatory response.

hemiplegia paralysis of one side of the body.

hemoptysis the coughing and spitting up of blood.

hemorrhage bleeding from a ruptured blood vessel externally or internally.

hiatal hernia a protrusion of a portion of the stomach through the esophageal hiatus of the diaphragm.

homeostenosis gradual decremental changes in the functional capacity of the body systems.

hospice a specialized program for terminally ill persons that emphasizes pain relief and comfort measures.

hospital-acquired pneumonia pneumonia, virulent in nature, with gram-negative microorganisms likely to be involved, acquired in a hospital environment.

hypercapnia an elevated $PaCO_2$.

hypochlorohydria an abnormally small amount of hydrochloric acid in the stomach.

hypothalamus the portion of the brain that activates and controls body temperature, among other things.

hypothermia abnormally low body temperature, <93°F.

hypoxemia abnormally low arterial oxygen tension; low PaO_2.

hypoxia deficiency of oxygen in the tissues.

idiopathic referring to a disease or condition for which the cause is unknown.

immunodeficient an abnormal inadequacy of the immune system.

immunological theory the immune system breaks down over time and there is an associated loss of cells in the thymic cortex.

institutionalization placing a person or a patient in an institution, usually in long-term care.

intima (tunica intima) the innermost layer of the wall of a vein or artery.

ischemia inadequate blood flow to a part of the body as a result of constriction or blockage of a blood vessel.

ischemic heart disease heart disease that is caused by an inadequate blood supply to the myocardium.

kyphosis an excessive outward curvature of the spine, also called *hunchback*.

kyphoscoliosis both a posterior and a lateral curvature of the spine.

lamina propria submucosal layer of the tracheobronchial tree.

life expectancy an average number of years remaining from a set point.

life review the psychological process of assessing one's life over time.

life span the maximum possible length of life for a species.

living will a legal statement outlining treatments the individual does not want (e.g., intubation, ventilator care) at the end of life.

locus of control location of one's personal control, either internal, external, or somewhere in between.

longitudinal research a research methodology where the same people are tested repeatedly over the course of years and their present results are compared to their own past performance.

manic impulsive behavior characterized by irritability and an inability to calm down, sometimes confounded with delusions of grandeur.

mechanoreceptor a sensory nerve cell activated by mechanical stimuli such as touch, pressure, sound, and muscular contractions.

media (tunica media) the middle layer of the wall of a vein or artery, composed of smooth muscle and elastic fibers.

multi-infarct dementia mental deterioration caused by a series of small strokes (infarcts); dementia characterized by a stepwise downward progression.

neoplasms any new or abnormal growth, benign or malignant, in which there is uncontrollable cell multiplication.

old old those 85 years of age or older.

organic disorders mental problems with an underlying physical cause, such as Alzheimer's disease, stroke or other brain trauma, Parkinson's disease, Pick's disease, Creutzfeld-Jacob syndrome, or brain tumor; the term is usually associated with dementing conditions.

orthopnea breathlessness or difficult breathing that is relieved by sitting in an upright or semivertical position.

osteoporosis a disease characterized by a reduction in the quantity of bone. It is a common manifestation of bone abnormality in older adults.

paranoid afflicted with suspicious, irrational beliefs.

paraphrenia delusional disorders in later life, but unlike schizophrenia, with an otherwise intact personality and mental structure.

paroxysmal nocturnal dyspnea difficulty in breathing in a recumbent position, such as sleeping at night, usually associated with congestive heart failure and pulmonary edema.

Patient Self-Determination Act federal legislation that, since 1991, has required health care programs and institutions to review life and death care options with newly-admitted patients.

pharmacodynamics relating to drug action.

pharmacokinetics relating to drug movement within the body.

polycythemia an increase in the total amount of red blood cells in the blood.

polypharmacy multiple drug use.

protein bound bound in plasma to the protein albumin and not biologically active.

pulsus paradoxus an exaggeration of the normal variation in pulse volume that occurs with respirations.

rate of living theory a simplistic theory of aging that posits that the length of life is related to the rate of metabolism; thus, tortoises outlive shrews.

rectangular survival curve a graph representing the trend for more and more people to survive childhood and midlife and live into old age.

sensorium the part of the consciousness associated with intellectual functioning.

septum a wall or portion that serves to separate or divide a body space or cavity.

slow code the practice of waiting a period of time before calling for CPR, which makes death a more certain outcome.

social death   the lowest end of a social worth continuum wherein the individual is treated mechanically, more like a thing than a person; comatose and demented patients are often socially dead long before they are physically dead.

social worth   an assignment of social value to people who are seen as more important and consequently seem to get better care than those at the bottom of the social ladder.

somatic mutation theory   genetic mutations caused by exposure to the environment, especially atomic radiation, are responsible for the aging process.

spend-down   depletion of one's assets to a point where Medicaid must pay for nursing home costs.

thrombus   a blood clot.

tortuous   twisted, having many curves and turns.

t-PA   tissue plasminogen activator, a clot-dissolving substance.

Trendelenburg   position in which the legs and feet are elevated and the head is lowered.

venostasis   a disorder characterized by an abnormally slow flow of blood through the veins.

wear and tear theory   the concept that biological aging is simply the process of tissues wearing out over time.

INDEX